Fundamentals of Epidemiology

Fundamentals of Epidemiology

An Instruction Manual

Donald R. Peterson, M.D.
David B. Thomas, M.D.
University of Washington

Lexington Books
D.C. Heath and Company
Lexington, Massachusetts
Toronto

Library of Congress Cataloging in Publication Data

Peterson, Donald Richard, 1921–
    Fundamentals of epidemiology.

    Includes index.
    1. Epidemiology. I. Thomas, David Bartlett, 1937–   joint author.
II. Title.
RA651.P48   614.4   77-11244
ISBN 0-669-01901-1

Fourth printing, April 1983

Published simultaneously in Canada

Printed in the United States of America

International Standard Book Number: 0-669-01901-1

Library of Congress Catalog Card Number: 77-11244

Contents

List of Figures

List of Tables

Preface

This manual is designed to serve as a means of self-instruction in fundamentals of epidemiology. It is intended as an introduction to the subject, and therefore the material presented is limited in scope. It differs from other texts in that the entire material is organized around a single theme, disease rates, a device adopted in an attempt to provide a cohesive presentation of the topic. The objectives of this manual are:

1. To impart knowledge of epidemiology as a discipline of learning and a field of practice;
2. To provide experience in applying epidemiologic principles to the solution of specific problems;
3. To enhance skill in critically evaluating professional medical literature.

References to problems occur at intervals throughout the text; there are eleven problems in all. Students are encouraged to answer the questions posed in each problem *in writing* before referring to the answers that appear at the end of the book.

A set of twenty multiple-choice examination questions is also included.

Acknowledgments

This manual was originally conceived and written during the tenure of one of the authors (Donald R. Peterson) as visiting lecturer in the Department of Social and Preventive Medicine, University of Malaya. Professor W. Danaraj (now deceased) generously provided necessary staff and physical resources. Miss Yap Mei Lin typed the entire first draft from handwritten copy, following which, after radical revision of the original account, she patiently retyped and proofread the entire manuscript. Several departmental faculty members consulted during the preparation of this volume offered useful suggestions, including Associate Professors Paul C.Y. Chen (now Professor) and P. Arumanayagam and Lecturers Lillian Lau and Teoh Soon Teong.

Subsequently, suggestions from students and faculty, at the University of Washington and elsewhere, too numerous to mention individually, resulted in further revisions. We gratefully acknowledge our debt to all who have aided us in preparing this manual.

Introduction

Epidemiology has proved to be difficult to define concisely yet comprehensively; those who have attempted the task have found colleagues quick to criticize their effort. One such individual, apparently in a fit of frustration, concluded: "Epidemiology is what an epidemiologist does."

Dictionaries have defined epidemiology simply as "that branch of medicine which deals with epidemics" or "the science of epidemics." Etymologically, the word derives from *epi*, upon; *demos*, people; and *logia*, knowledge.

Some definers have portrayed epidemiology in broad, short strokes, as in the following:

The science of the mass phenomenon of disease.

The study of the laws and factors governing the occurrence of disease or abnormality in a population group.

The study of the distribution and determinants of disease in man.

The art and science of disease occurrence.

Epidemiology is medical ecology.

Another set of definitions has an expository character, as in the following:

The science which concerns itself with the natural history of disease as it is expressed in groups of persons related by some common factors of age, sex, race, location, or occupation as distinct from development of disease in individuals.

That field of medical science which is concerned with the relationship of the various factors and conditions which determine the frequencies and distributions of an infectious process, disease, or a physiological state in a community.

Epidemiology is concerned with searching out and understanding the factors relating to the occurrence and distribution of disease in the population, studying the sick and the well in relation to each other and the environment.

The art and science of identifying factors responsible for differing frequency distributions of health-related phenomena in human society in order to devise and test ways and means for their control.

A simplistic expository definition, phrased in descriptive pronouns, covers the major points of the preceding ones:

The professional discipline concerned with describing health related phenomena in human populations, specifically *how much* with respect to *when, where,* and *who* for the purpose of explaining *why* such phenomena occur and *what* can be done about them.

This definition can be phrased more succinctly: *Epidemiology is the study of the distribution, determinants, and deterrents of disease in human populations.*

Somewhat contrary to the foregoing, Fox has observed that:

Epidemiology is not the proprietor of a well-defined and homogeneous body of knowledge as in the case with a basic or pure science such as chemistry. Rather, epidemiology is a discipline which has evolved relatively specialized methods for investigating disease causation and bringing to bear, according to needs of the moment, specific knowledge and special skills from many other sciences. With some justice epidemiology has been called a method rather than a independent science.*

Epidemiologists engage in a wide variety of professional pursuits directed at a broad range of health problems, and their work inevitably involves quantification of health-related phenomena in populations by means of disease rates or some comparable measure. The basic elements or fundamentals of epidemiology therefore include those concepts and principles which pertain to the composition of disease rates, the processes of acquiring their components, the interpretation of results obtained with such instruments, and the uses to which they can be put.

*J.P. Fox, C.E. Hall, and L.R. Elveback, *Epidemiology: Man and Disease* (Toronto: The Macmillan Company, 1970), p. 10.

Disease Rates

Incidence and Prevalence

Two types of rates are used in epidemiology. These are termed *incidence* and *prevalence.*

The incidence of a disease is the proportion of people in a population under study or observation that develop the disease of interest during a defined period of time. Disease incidence is a measure of disease *risk*, and is of utmost importance for epidemiologic purposes.

The prevalence of a disease or attribute is simply the proportion of people in a population under study or observation that have the condition of interest at a particular point in time. Of interest to epidemiologists and clinicians are both the prevalence of various conditions in different populations, and the prevalence of a variety of factors that may be related to disease occurrence.

Rate Components

In principle, then, disease rates are simple arithmetic expressions denoting a population fraction or proportion. They consist of a numerator, a denominator, and a coefficient (termed a *rate base*), as shown in the following:

$$\text{Disease rate} = \frac{\text{numerator}}{\text{denominator}} \times \text{a base} =$$

$$\frac{\text{Number of persons who develop or have a particular disease during a specified time interval or at a point in time}}{\text{Total number of persons comprising the population to which the persons with a particular disease belonged during the same time frame}} \times \text{some multiple of } 10.$$

Because disease rate by definition is a fraction (or proportion), it is also

1

important to note that the persons comprising the numerator should also appear in the denominator.

$$\text{Disease rate} = \frac{\text{diseased}}{\text{diseased} + \text{nondiseased}} \times \text{base}$$

Rate Base

As a general rule, in choosing a rate base one selects some multiple of ten that will yield a computed rate value that equals or exceeds unity. For example, if the quotient obtained by dividing the number of people with a particular disease in a certain community by the total number of residents of that community equaled 0.0052, a rate base of 1,000 would yield a rate of 5.2 per 1,000 population. Should one choose instead to use a rate base of 10,000, the rate value would be 52 per 10,000 population. If the proportion affected were relatively large (for example, in excess of 0.1), a rate base of 100 might provide the most cogent population unit for referencing the rate value. In practice, the use of a rate base of 100, which expresses disease frequency in percentage, usually results from focal (sharply localized) epidemics involving a circumscribed subset of the population that is susceptible to a highly communicable disease-producing agent or some widely distributed toxic substance to which many are exposed.

Rates for uncommon conditions are conventionally expressed in population units of 100,000 or 1,000,000, depending upon the calculated quotient value.

For some commonly encountered health-related phenomena, a uniform or conventional rate base has been adopted. For example, mortality rates—the rates of dying from any and all causes—are traditionally expressed in population units of 1,000. In the event that custom is ignored, it is a simple matter to convert a nonconventional to a conventional rate base by moving the decimal point in one direction or the other in order to put the rate value into familiar perspective. From the foregoing, the rate base emerges as a useful but noncritical appendage with respect to how well a disease rate reflects what transpires relative to disease occurrence in populations.

Rate Denominators

Periodic enumerations of populations under government auspices constitute one common source of information for denominators. Because of the inherent value of such demographic information to business executives, public administrators (including those in health agencies), and many others, an official census of a population ordinarily includes a wealth of subclassifications that cater to these special interests.

The ubiquitous role that age and sex play in human affairs of every description, including politics and health, has long been recognized; an official census, therefore, invariably includes figures that detail the age and sex composition of the population.

The *population pyramid* is a conventional way of depicting the age and sex distribution of a population. Figure 1 illustrates how radically populations can differ with respect to their age-sex composition. The data on which the Malay population pyramid is based came from the 1970 population and housing census of Malaysia, conducted on August 26, 1970. According to this census the total Malay population in West Malaysia on that date numbered 4,672,822; age was recorded as unknown for 12,561 males and 11,884 females—0.5 percent in each case, a negligible proportion. The Washington State material came from the 1970 decennial United States census of Washington State, conducted on April 1, 1970; the total comprised 3,409,169 residents of Washington State on that date, with an age reported for each one.

These two populations, of similar size and enumerated at about the same time, exhibit salient differences in their age and sex distribution patterns. The broad-based shape of the Malay graph is typical of rural populations disadvantaged by less than adequate living conditions. Life expectancy is low, births are numerous, and the proportion of individuals in each age group markedly decreases with advancing years. By contrast, Washingtonians live in a highly developed industrial/agrarian society, with a lower birth rate and fewer people dying until old age. The age-sex profile is therefore more columnar than pyramidal, with a proportionately large segment of the total number making up the older age groups.

In addition to age and sex tabulations, an official census in the United States usually provides data on such items as occupation of head of household, income level of households, years of schooling of individuals, quality of housing, and marital status of individuals—to mention a few demographic variables that can be used as disease rate denominators if an occasion warrants. The variables mentioned are usually tabulated according to geographic units and subunits, that is, nation, states, counties, cities, towns, rural areas, and specially designated census tracts, as well as blocks.

A decennial or other population census provides a profile of the population stream in cross section at a point in time. Viewed as a sequence, consecutive cross sections mirror the extent to which a geographically circumscribed population, in its course through time, is fed by births and immigration and bled by deaths and emigration, with corresponding shifts in composition. Each profile may be likened to a snapshot or still photograph of a continuum of change that only a continuous inventory analogous to a cinematic recording would accord—a patently impractical accomplishment on a nationwide scale.

Denominator figures for times between or beyond census takings must therefore be estimated by interpolation or extrapolation, respectively. Because

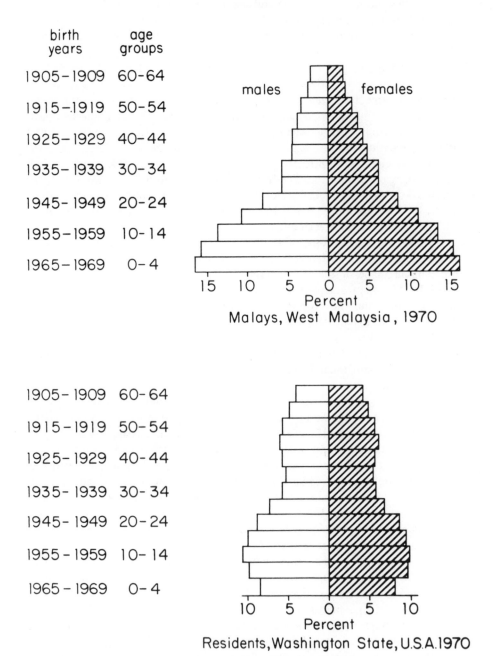

Figure 1. Distribution of Two Populations by Age and Sex

births and deaths are generally recorded and tabulated on a monthly or annual basis, incremental or decremental adjustments for these factors help in such population estimations. However, if considerable immigration or emigration takes place between census periods, estimations can miss the mark significantly, with obvious consequences for calculated disease rates.

For the reason just cited, as well as others, intercensal surveys based on population samples may be conducted to update certain demographic information if its importance warrants the rather considerable expense that such enterprise entails.

Other official sources of denominator data, which on occasion can be useful for disease rate denominators, include live birth registrations, persons listed on tax rolls, school enrollment figures, and so forth. The sources mentioned possess the distinct advantage of being collected at least annually—a feature that diminishes the uncertainty associated with denominator material collected at less frequent intervals.

Nonofficial information of a demographic sort will sometimes accommodate a special epidemiological purpose. Personnel files, life insurance company records, and lists of subscribers to health insurance plans or other essential services exemplify this sort of ready-made denominator material.

When the need of the moment extends beyond existing resources for obtaining denominators, the alternatives include: (1) collecting special information from all persons in the population of interest; (2) collecting such information from a probability sample of that population; or (3) resorting to "samples of convenience," which will be considered in a subsequent section.

The fidelity with which a disease rate mirrors actual happenings obviously depends upon the precision with which individuals constituting both the numerator and denominator are enumerated. Of these two components, errors in the denominator produce less distortion of rates, in most instances, than do errors in the numerator. However, errors in rates due to faulty denominators can and do occur. For example, cancer death rates for young male blacks were found to exceed those for whites, but older whites had higher rates. The reason for this peculiar observation became apparent when it was discovered that young male blacks were substantially undernumerated by the official census.

The Disease Spectrum Concept

Enumeration of cases for inclusion in the numerator component of a disease rate is a complicated process. A definition of a case must be clearly formulated; then, individuals meeting the criteria for a case must be detected, counted, and characterized by variables of interest. Both case definition and case detection are strongly influenced by variation in the way diseases are manifest. Comprehension of this concept of a disease spectrum is thus critical to an understanding of disease rates. Figure 2 depicts the disease spectrum concept schematically.

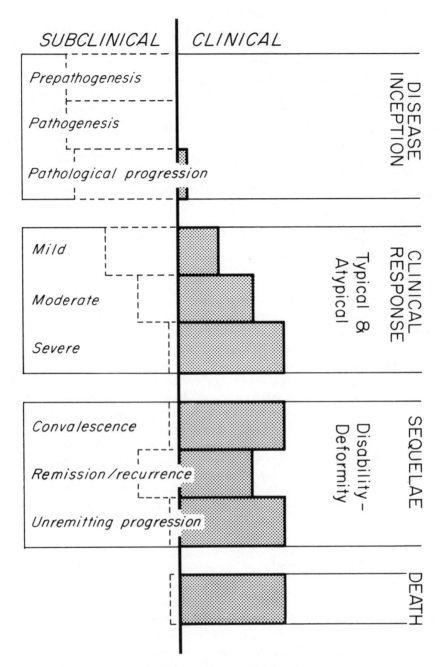

Figure 2. The Disease Spectrum

In the figure, the vertical bars represent portions of the disease spectrum and the dark horizontal line divides each of these into clinically apparent and subclinical parts. The extent to which disease exists as subclinical will vary in relation to the state of progression, the severity of response, and the devices the physician or epidemiologist uses to detect or diagnosis it.

Some diseases exhibit a *prodrome* (nondistinguishing symptoms or signs), which precedes the development of a clinically recognizable *syndrome*; occasionally, a single *pathognomonic* sign or symptom heralds the presence of disease. The period of disease inception may vary in length from seconds (in the case of injury by violence, for example) to years (as in diabetes mellitus or mental illness). The end of the disease inception period marks the beginning of the clinical response phase.

The time of illness onset plays a crucial role in epidemiological strategy and tactics. When the departure from a previous health state is abrupt, and therefore clearly demarcated in time by exact date or even hour of the day, the fact of disease onset can be handily established. There are some diseases, however, whose onset is insidious and therefore can be expressed only as lying within some relatively long time interval gauged in weeks or months rather than days or hours.

Just as individuals differ in appearance, personality, and other attributes, so do they differ in their response to a disease process with respect to severity of disease expression. Furthermore, people will differ with respect to symptoms and signs that indicate manifest disease. For any given disease, a majority of patients will have symptoms and signs that are typical of the disease from a clinical point of view. A few individuals, however, can be expected to evidence atypical symptoms and signs.

Atypical clinical responses result not only from endogenous influences, such as age, genetic endowment, and innate but partial resistance, but also from exogenous factors, such as intervention with therapeutic modalities that, by their action, either mask or exaggerate certain features of the clinical response. Concomitant disease, poor nutritional status, dose or degree of exposure to a disease agent, or other influences may also alter the clinical picture.

Obviously, disease processes that usually produce uniform clinical manifestations, that is, typical syndromes, will afford a more homogeneous collection of individuals for disease rate numerators than those that entail diagnostic uncertainty.

The third sector of the diagram in Figure 2 subtends the various sequelae that can ensue following the phase of clinical response. Fortunately, many of the ills to which humans are heir subside within a relatively short period of time after onset; the clinical phase shades into convalescence almost without notice, following which the affected individual enjoys restoration to his prior state of health—perhaps better in some ways than before, insofar as his appreciation of the "gift of health" is concerned. On the other hand, an affected individual may be left with a certain residual of the disease experience.

The sequelae of a disease encompass many expressions that can be utilized epidemiologically for qualifying disease rate numerators. Surgical scars, deformity of internal organs visualized radiographically, permanent physical or mental disability, sensory or motor dysfunction, immunological changes, or morphological change (deformity) may, in certain situations, prove useful as markers that can be used to identify persons for disease rate numerator purposes.

The diagram also indicates that some diseases may exhibit more than a single clinical response phase, with periods of remission alternating with periods of recurrence; the underlying disease process does not subside completely but remains dormant during remissions. Some diseases, after running their course, confer immunity to recurrence, which may be lifelong in duration or last a substantial length of time. On the other hand, there are diseases which may be contracted *de novo*, again and again, under propitious circumstances (gonorrhea, for example).

Unfortunately, some diseases, once established, do not subside; affected persons remain chronically ill, with little hope of recovery. Still other diseases produce a prolonged illness episode that progresses to the point of deterioration of the individual; in such situations the distinction between the clinical response phase and the sequelae phase becomes blurred, as shown in the disease spectrum diagram.

Finally, diseases vary in their propensity to destroy human life. Some are totally benign in this respect, whereas others, once incurred, are inevitably fatal. Between these extremes lie a host of diseases for which a lethal outcome has varying probabilities. Strange as it may seem, some disease processes remain subclinical throughout their course of evolution, and their presence becomes dramatically manifest by the event of death without warning, which occurs suddenly and unexpectedly.

As presented in general outline on these pages, the disease spectrum concept emerges as a kaleidoscopic array of options that may be exercised for disease rate numerator classification purposes. In attacking a particular disease problem, specific knowledge is fitted within this conceptual frame as appropriate in order to distinguish those qualitative aspects that can be utilized epidemiologically. Much of the knowledge that is pertinent to the disease spectrum concept must be culled from other fields of health-related scientific endeavor—clinical medicine, physiology, biochemistry, microbiology, immunology, radiology, pathology, and so forth. The depth of such knowledge determines the extent to which one can employ the disease spectrum concept to provide a comprehensive perspective of a specific disease in the various guises and disguises in which it appears among the diversity of individuals who comprise a population. The lack of such knowledge may preclude an epidemiological attack altogether or limit disease rate calculations to only gross approximations; many mental disorders defy close epidemiological scrutiny because of diagnostic and prognostic uncertainties.

It should be noted that, from a practical point of view, identification on a community-wide basis of every individual in every phase of the spectrum of a specific disease is seldom possible. Usually one selects one or more portions from the entire spectrum that suit specific needs.

The common contagious disease of childhood, mumps (epidemic parotitis, infectious sialitis), provides an instructive example of the disease spectrum concept. The period of disease inception begins with an individual's encounter for the first time with the etiologic agent of the disease, a virus of the myxovirus group that is pathogenic only for humans. Viral infection results from exposure to one or more other individuals who are at that stage in the evolution of the disease during which virus shedding via one or more *portals of exit* takes place. Salivary gland secretions from such individuals are heavily charged with virus. During talking, laughing, coughing, and sneezing, tiny liquid droplets (*aerosols*) or their dried residua (*droplet nuclei*), which contain the viable infective agent, are expelled. Some are inadvertently inhaled or ingested by a susceptible individual. Those virus particles which gain access to the new host through a *portal of entry* that exposes them to the type of tissue cell for which they have special affinity (*tropism*) penetrate tissue cells, replicate, invade adjacent cells, eventually become blood-borne (*viremia*), and spread throughout the body. This usually transpires without any outward manifestation except perhaps a low-grade fever and lassitude during the viremic stage. When pathogenesis reaches a point when one or more organs (*target organs*) become structurally and/or functionally disordered, symptoms and signs materialize.

The phase of disease inception, or *incubation period*, ranges from 12 to 26 days for mumps, and is most commonly about 18 days. For a day or two prior to the onset of overt illness and for several days thereafter during the state of clinical response, the affected individual unwittingly serves as a *vector of disease transmission* to others; in this way the virus is propagated by person-to-person spread and thereby perpetuated in nature.

The stage of clinical response consists primarily of the classical mumps syndrome of fever, malaise, dysphagia, and bulging jaws bilaterally. Some individuals experience salivary gland swelling on one side only. A few individuals respond atypically with symptoms and signs indicating involvement of such sites as the meninges, testes, ovaries, or pancreas (sometimes accompanied by a short-term diabetic state). These may occur with or without parotid or other salivary gland inflammation. Other infected persons will have no symptoms or signs.

Responses from 117 medical students to a questionnaire concerning their personal experience with mumps illustrate the variability just described. Among the 68 students who were reasonably certain that they had had mumps (usually during early childhood), 16 indicated that they had experienced unilateral parotid swelling, compared to 49 with bilateral involvement. Two students stated that they had no parotid swelling but rather submaxillary salivary gland hypertrophy. One student reported that he had mumps on three separate occasions, with bilateral parotid swelling once and unilateral involvement twice; probably only one of these episodes was actually mumps. Twelve of the 117 students were uncertain whether or not they had had mumps. The remainder (26 students) confidently denied a history of mumps illness; 10 of the 26 recalled that a brother or sister with whom they lived had had mumps. These 10 very likely were inapparently infected (subclinical mumps). Only one student reported meningoencephalitis as a sequel to bilateral parotid involvement. None recalled gonadal involvement. Because sequelae occur mostly among those infected after puberty, these results are consonant with onset of disease during early childhood.

The effects of late-onset mumps have been quantified by a review of records of the Mayo Clinic for the period 1935-1974. Among 1310 cases of mumps, 121 developed orchitis. The median age of the entire group of mumps cases was 8 years; however, the median age of the 121 who experienced orchitis was 29 years.

For most who contract mumps infection, an uneventful and short convalescence, which follows the state of clinical response, ends the experience. For an unfortunate few, mumps virus infection leaves the host with permanent disabling residua, including sterility, deafness, paralysis, mental retardation, and perhaps a later predisposition to diabetes mellitus. Occasionally, this disease eventuates in death. Those who survive acquire immunity to subsequent infection with mumps virus, which is ordinarily lifelong in duration. The immune state can be identified by serological tests that measure the level (concentration) of mumps-specific antibody.

The serological testing of groups of people with and without a medical history of mumps (prior to the advent of mumps virus vaccine) has revealed that about one-third of those with naturally acquired antibody have a negative history of clinical mumps. In other words, clinically inapparent cases account for 33 percent of total infections. A disease rate numerator based on clinical mumps cases is thus an underestimate of the number of infected persons.

Idiopathic epilepsy provides another example of the disease spectrum. The adjective *idiopathic* denotes ignorance of the etiology and pathogenesis of this disease.

The period of inception of epilepsy represents a void that one hopes might eventually be filled. It is clear, however, that some underlying disturbance in cerebral physiology, which erupts spontaneously and sporadically, produces the classic grand mal seizure.

Typically, those with this disease first experience a premonition that something is about to happen (this is termed an *aura*); next, they utter an involuntary cry as they collapse and become rigid because of tonic spasm of the extensor muscles; clonic or jerking movements of the body supervene, during which involuntary defecation and micturition occur. Seizures usually last a matter of minutes, after which the victim's senses are obtunded and he yearns for sleep.

The first seizure experienced by a person may be the last, in which case there is only a single clinical response phase. Other people experience seizures of varying degrees of severity, rarely or frequently, over their lifetimes, thereby exhibiting recurrences and remissions. Those with frequent and severe seizure patterns eventually accumulate sufficient brain damage as a result of repeated hypoxic episodes to experience such sequelae as psychosis, mental deterioration, and eventually death. Obviously, such unfortunates also experience more than their share of trauma from such things as falling and tongue biting. Effective anticonvulsant medications are capable of preventing or modifying epileptic seizures in many individuals.

The next topic, disease incidence, is predicated on the disease spectrum concept.

Disease Incidence

We have seen that the term *disease incidence* denotes disease events that can be categorized with respect to time of onset. Conventionally, time of onset is taken to be the beginning of the clinical response state of the disease. Accordingly, incident cases of disease are often defined as "new" cases on the implied premise that such individuals were experiencing their first encounter with a particular disease. However, this interpretation ignores the fact that incidence has a broader connotation—that of designating a departure from a previous state of health. One can therefore speak quite properly of the incidence of first, second, and so forth, attacks of a particular disease, the incidence of recurrences, the incidence of remissions, and the incidence of deaths. The basis for such classification rests on the condition that such events can be demarcated on a time scale.

For many diseases the time of onset of the symptom that appears first suffices as an onset marker. If, however, the first symptom begins insidiously as a vague subjective feeling of unwellness, then the first salient symptom, preferably one that can be verified objectively by a cognitive sign, can be used for establishing onset time. For example, the onset of nausea that usually precedes vomiting is often difficult to relate to a precise time, whereas the onset of the act of vomiting generally poses no difficulty in the same respect. (Problem 1 should prove instructive at this point.)

If the advent of an entire syndrome cannot be precisely specified as occurring at a specific hour or on a particular day because of the gradualness of the development of signs and symptoms, then a coarser time scale (weeks or months) or an associated event may provide a suitable approximation. The date of first absence from school or work, the date of first medical consultation, the date of diagnosis, the date of first hospitalization, or the date of official notification of a reportable disease have been used as surrogates for actual onset time on occasion.

The frequency with which disease occurs in a population during successive time intervals provides a measure of disease dynamics by which the waxing or waning of disease occurrence over time can be distinguished from a steady state. *Epidemics* are defined simply as any substantial increase in disease incidence over the usual incidence level—sometimes referred to as the *endemic* level. If a particular disease has been absent from a community for a period of time, the occurrence of just a few cases might warrant the label epidemic (the appellation disease *outbreak* is also used). On the other hand, if the usual frequency were appreciable, a substantial number of cases would have to accrue before the distinction "epidemic" would apply. The term *pandemic* refers to a worldwide epidemic.

The ability to distinguish epidemic from endemic disease occurrence obviously depends upon an appropriate bookkeeping system for entering the date of onset as well as other pertinent items of information so that disease incidence patterns in relation to calendar time can be ascertained and utilized.

Epidemic Curves

If shifts in population size or composition occur during a time period when disease incidence is under scrutiny, the necessity for calculations of rates in order to take into account the demographic changes is obvious. Over a short term, however, when the population from which incident cases emerge can be considered stable, simple enumeration of incident cases themselves can be used to epidemiological advantage.

When dealing with acute diseases, by plotting the frequency of incident cases according to hour, day, week, or month of onset one obtains a graphic depiction of the *epidemic curve* in the form of a *frequency histogram*. Figure 3 illustrates an epidemic curve constructed to show the number of incident cases of gastroenteritis in consecutive one-hour time segments. The onset time was taken as the hour during which explosive diarrhea began.

The distribution of incident cases shown in Figure 3 is unimodal. This means it has one mode, or point of increased frequency of cases. Also, the range of times of onset is scaled in hours and is relatively narrow. One implication of such a pattern is that the afflicted individuals may have experienced a common exposure, at a single point in time, to some disease-producing agent and that the variability in time of disease onset reflects individual differences in clinical response. For some diseases due to bacteria or toxins, such variability may also be dose-related, with those most exposed to the disease-producing agent becoming ill sooner than those who had a lesser exposure.

For certain diseases produced by infectious agents or toxins, the length of the disease inception state (incubation period) consistently lies within relatively narrow limits. This fact not only may help confirm the diagnosis, but also may

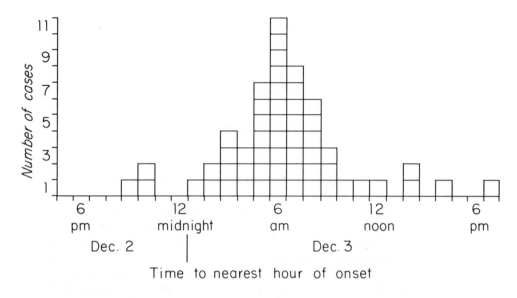

Figure 3. Frequency Histogram, Incident Cases, Gastroenteritis

identify a point in time when a common exposure took place. Figure 3 portrays an outbreak of gastroenteritis produced by *Clostridium perfringens*. The incubation period range was 7 to 24 hours following exposure, with the greatest frequency at 12 hours. These results are typical of food-associated outbreaks produced by this organism.

If the frequency distribution of incident cases depicted histographically over time has a wide range or exhibits two or more waves (modes), one can surmise either that transmission is accomplished via person-to-person spread, or that persons are exposed to one or more nonhuman sources (air, water, contaminated articles (fomites), arthroped vectors, and so forth) over a period of time.

For a disease propagated by person-to-person contact, the interval between peaks of the epidemic curve indicates the length of the *generation time*, which usually approximates the induction period of the particular disease.

Figure 4 illustrates an incidence pattern compatible with person-to-person disease propagation. The interval between the successive generations of cases corresponds well with the known incubation period of chickenpox (varicella). In this instance, it seems likely that the first group of cases occurred as a result of exposure to a single *index case*, and that subsequent waves of cases resulted from exposures to one or more infectious children in the first wave. Cases that occurred as a result of exposure to the index case are termed *secondary cases*. This term is frequently used in describing disease outbreaks in families. (Problem 2 deals with an epidemic curve.)

As long as the assumption of a stable denominator holds, other temporal

14

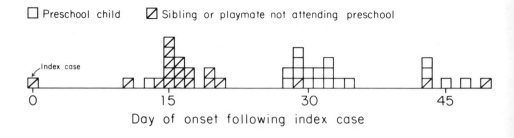

□ Preschool child   ☑ Sibling or playmate not attending preschool

Day of onset following index case

Figure 4. Chickenpox Cases, April–June 1971

patterns can also be studied from simple frequency distributions of incident cases. The distribution of cases by day of the week of disease onset, irrespective of actual date, may prove useful in investing certain health-related phenomena, such as motor vehicle accidents, for example. Many diseases exhibit seasonal swings in incidence, readily perceived from frequency tabulations of cases by month of onset.

Plotting incident cases on a map to elucidate their location in relation to potential sources of etiologic agents is also a useful technique that does not involve computation of rates.

Disease Prevalence

Disease prevalence deals with the sum of individuals who, at some point in time or during some period of time, can be classified as diseased, irrespective of the time of onset of the disease in question. With respect to the disease spectrum concept, prevalent cases at a point in time would include not only individuals in the clinical response phase but also those in the portion labeled sequelae. Deaths, remissions, and cures, of course, would be excluded.

The enumeration of persons classified as prevalent cases of some disease at a point in time yields an estimate of the *point prevalence* for that disease; in this connection the point is usually a given day (or perhaps several days if the ascertainment process takes longer than a day to accomplish). The term *disease prevalence* usually signifies a point estimate. A *period prevalence* estimate results from a point estimate at the beginning of some specified time interval to which incident cases occurring during the interval are added so as to comprise all cases extant within the period.

A prevalence figure based on all existing cases of a particular disease provides a measure of the total burden of that disease on a population.

The needs of the moment will dictate which portion of the disease spectrum will provide the appropriate prevalence rates. The prevalence of tuberculosis, for example, can be expressed in several ways. A prevalence based on persons hospitalized for this disease would interest those with responsiblity for providing facilities for the long-term medical care that is often necessary for the more severe forms of this chronic infectious process. Milder cases may simply be restricted to their homes while receiving long-term chemotherapy to arrest the disease process and render them noninfectious.

The prevalence of individuals with chest X-ray evidence of tuberculosis can be dichotomized into those with evidence of recently acquired disease and those with older lesions at various stages of progression or regression. The number of individuals with recently acquired disease for whom prompt and adequate treatment holds a promise of complete health restoration, added to those on home treatment for symptomatic, though mild, disease, amplifies the prevalence picture. Finally, persons with positive tuberculin skin test reactions, who have no clinical or radiographic evidence of tuberculosis, comprise another prevalence category. The positive test as a solo finding indicates infection with the etiologic agent (*Mycobacterium tuberculosis*), which has not evolved sufficiently to produce a radiographic lesion or symptoms and signs. Individuals so stigmatized may be either treated or examined periodically for evidence of disease progression. Within this mosaic of prevalences, another of singular importance can be dissected out, namely, individuals whose disease, at whatever stage of evolution, might render them infectious to others by virtue of the presence of viable *M. tuberculosis* in their sputum. The prevalence of such persons, or those likely to become sources of infection, reveals the size of the human *reservoir of infection* that will contribute to the subsequent production of incident cases (newly acquired infection), among their contacts—obviously an important aspect for eventual control of the disease.

In the event that one or more nonhuman life forms are implicated as an infectious disease reservoir, the prevalence of infection among subhuman populations becomes a matter of epidemiological concern and importance. The aid of veterinarians, mammalogists, ornithologists, entomologists, and so forth, must be enlisted to work on the epizoology of the disease in question.

One can quantitate certain types of disability, irrespective of the diseases responsible, using prevalence rates. For example, many different diseases may culminate in disabling arthritis; it may suit some practical purpose (even commercial) to measure the prevalence of disabling arthritis from any cause rather than specific forms.

Many cancers exist for relatively long periods and can be detected in examinable tissues (skin, breast, uterine cervix) while in a quiescent or dormant state during their stage of disease inception. The prevalence of precursive cancer lesions has a considerable bearing on the success of attempts to control cancer incidence by early detection and extirpation.

Diseases that evoke an immunogenic response, such as the formation of specific antibody, can be investigated epidemiologically by measuring antibody prevalence in populations.

Incidence and Prevalence Rates

The disease rate numerator determines whether a rate reflects incidence or prevalence. If the numerator comprises the total number of persons classified as either incident cases or as prevalent cases, and the denominator includes the entire population, the resulting rate is referred to as a *crude rate*. The terms *overall* or *total* rate are also appropriate.

An overall disease incidence rate consists of the following components:

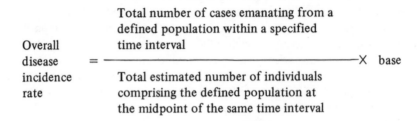

$$\text{Overall disease incidence rate} = \frac{\text{Total number of cases emanating from a defined population within a specified time interval}}{\text{Total estimated number of individuals comprising the defined population at the midpoint of the same time interval}} \times \text{base}$$

Mortality rates may serve as an index of disease incidence when a large proportion of people with the disease die from it within a relatively short time of onset. Mortality rates have an identical construction to that shown above, with deaths substituted for cases.

Similarly, an overall point prevalence rate can be defined as follows:

$$\text{Overall disease point prevalence rate} = \frac{\text{Total number of cases extant at some point in time in a defined population irrespective of time of onset}}{\text{Total number of individuals comprising the defined population at the same point in time}} \times \text{base}$$

Overall incidence and prevalence rates provide the basic measures for judging whether a specific disease occurs rarely, commonly, or somewhere in between—useful distinctions generally, but especially for vendors of health services, both curative and preventive, and for setting health teaching priorities. Overall rates also serve to indicate the extent to which diseases wax and wane over the long term (termed *secular trends*), either as the result of natural forces or those incurred by human behavior or environmental modification. Overall incidence or prevalence rates also provide a guide for evaluating efforts designed to prevent disease or to lessen the frequency of certain sequelae. Figure 5 shows the secular incidence trends of two diseases, syphilis and gonorrhea, which illustrate occurrence patterns over a time span exceeding 50 years. The marked rise in reported syphilis in the early 1930s no doubt is an artifact resulting from

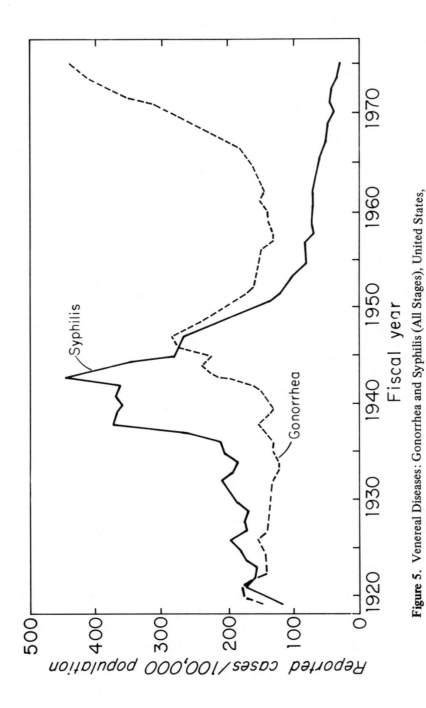

Figure 5. Venereal Diseases: Gonorrhea and Syphilis (All Stages), United States, 1919-1975

specific efforts at the national level to encourage case reporting. The super-imposed peak in the early 1940s, attended by a concommitant rise in gonorrhea, reflects the consequences of the social disruption occasioned by World War II. The decreased incidence of both diseases following the war years probably resulted not only from social restabilization but also from the widespread use of penicillin. *Treponema pallidum*, the agent responsible for syphilis, has remained sensitive to this antibiotic, whereas *Neisseria gonorrhoeae* has developed resistance. Antibiotic resistance, plus the changes in attitudes toward sex and in sex practices during the late 1960s and early 1970s, probably accounts for the continuing increase in gonorrhea incidence.

Figure 6 shows the secular mortality trends, separately for males and females, for three of the more common cancers. Both males and females exhibit a consistent, substantial downward trend in death from cancer of the stomach. Thus far, no one has explained why this has occurred, although changes in methods of food preservation that occurred during the period from 1930 to 1970 have been suggested as a possibility. The graph for males reveals a dramatic increase in deaths from lung cancer since 1930, which is primarily due to the marked increase in use of cigarettes since 1900. Female rates for lung cancer increased more slowly until 1965; since then they have risen as rapidly as did the male rates 35 years previously. This observation is consistent with the fact that women generally adopted the habit a number of years later than men. The secular trends of colon cancers show less striking variation in their pattern of occurrence over the four decades.

Disease duration and disease incidence determine disease prevalence. Under stable conditions with respect to incidence, and average disease duration, one can calculate any one of the three, if the other two are known, by appropriate transposition and substitution in the following algebraic expression: $P = I \times D$, where P stands for the point prevalence rate at the midpoint of a specified period, I denotes the overall incidence rate during the same period, and D indicates the average duration of the cases occurring during the period. Figure 7 illustrates the principle involved. In each year the midyear point prevalence consists of one case, with onset in the previous year and two in the current year. If the duration of each case were two years instead of one, as depicted, the line lengths would double and produce double the prevalence.

In the more usual event that the three measures are not stable, one may still impute the probable direction of change, even though the degree of change cannot be quantified. For example, if the disease incidence rate increases but the average duration remains unchanged, then the prevalence rate is bound to increase. If, on the other hand, a new treatment shortens the average disease duration, the prevalence rate will decrease, even though the incidence rate remains constant or even increases slightly. An effective life-saving drug, by forestalling the time of death of those who are chronically ill with a particular disease, may increase the disease prevalence rate by virtue of lengthening the

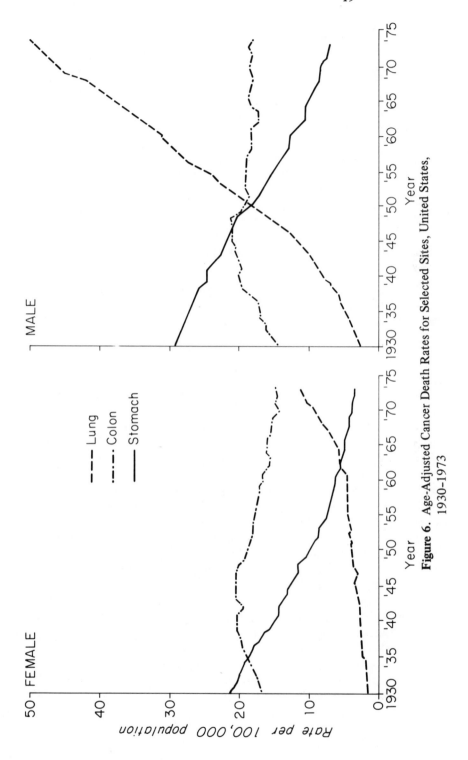

Figure 6. Age-Adjusted Cancer Death Rates for Selected Sites, United States, 1930-1973

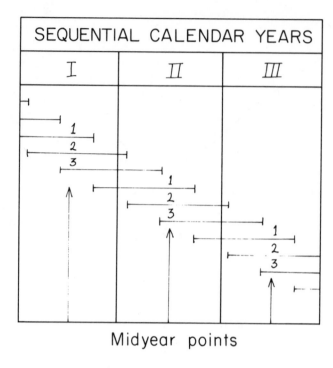

Figure 7. Scheme for Relating Incidence, Point Prevalence, and Duration

disease duration, even though the incidence rate of the disease does not change appreciably. If disease duration is fixed, on the average, then a decrease in the incidence rate will produce a decrease in the prevalence rate as well.

The *case fatality rate* (or case fatality ratio) is the proportion (or percentage) of cases of a particular disease that die as a result of the disease. This rate can be determined by following a group of cases for a defined period of time and observing how many die during that time period. The case fatality rate for cases of a disease that occur in a defined population can also be estimated by dividing the mortality rate by the incidence rate. The case fatality rate is an indicator of the severity of the disease. (Problem 3 deals with the calculation of incidence and prevalence rates and their interrelationships.)

Because populations may differ considerably in composition as well as size, overall disease incidence and prevalence rates provide rather gross estimates of disease occurrence. In order to probe within a population, rates must be computed for specific subsets, that is, age groups, the separate sexes, racial groups, groups exposed to specific substances, and so forth. Theoretically, specific rates for virtually any personal attribute can be computed; practically, specific rates are limited by the availability of appropriate numerator and denominator material.

The usual situation is that one has considerably more items of information concerning individuals comprising a disease rate numerator than for those making up the denominator; the limiting factor for the number of specific rates that can be computed for a particular disease is lack of demographic information. Rates can be made specific in a variety of ways to suit particular purposes. An overall incidence or prevalence rate for a particular disease is, by definition, *cause-specific*; if further elaborated by subdividing by sex, then the rates would be considered specific for both cause and sex; if subdivided still further by separation into certain age groups, the rates become specific for cause, sex, and age. The degree to which a disease rate can be made specific for different factors determines the depth to which populations can be probed epidemiologically. (Problem 4 deals with a number of commonly used conventional rates that have practical applications.)

The Disease Iceberg Concept

The iceberg metaphor has been and still is used extensively to describe various phenomena that have a proportionately large invisible component analagous to the four-fifths of an iceberg that is submerged and therefore invisible. With respect to disease rates, the disease iceberg concept dovetails with and complements the disease spectrum concept. The disease spectrum concept concerns the diversity of disease expression in a population, which is relevant for *qualitative* aspects of disease rate numerators. The iceberg concept, as will be shown, concerns the diversity (and perversity) of human behavior and institutions that bear on *quantitative* aspects of disease rate numerators, that is, completeness of ascertainment of cases.

When calculating disease rates in a population, a disease rate numerator should contain only those individuals within the population with the disease—no more, no less. This ideal, though seldom realized completely, can be approximated sufficiently for practical purposes if certain elements that have a bearing on quantification are appreciated and taken into account, namely:

1. the extent to which people in a community utilize the scientifically oriented medical establishment;
2. the extent to which physicians, as an integral part of the medical establishment, correctly diagnose their patients; and
3. the extent to which correctly diagnosed cases can be ascertained on a community-wide scale.

Some individuals, when faced with a health problem, turn to unconventional or noninstitutionalized resources, such as family, friends, pharmacists, clergymen, or quacks. Others, more stoical perhaps, rely solely upon themselves and confide in no one. Such behavior undoubtedly occurs most frequently in relation to diseases that are believed to be self-limiting, are of mild to moderate severity with respect to discomfort or disability, and are not perceived as a threat to life or limb. Shame, fear, or lack of faith in the medical profession deter some people from seeking consultation, even with severe discomfort or disability or, surprisingly, even with a premonition that their affliction may be lethal.

This behavior probably occurs to some extent with every disease, but for some diseases it occurs to such an extent that quantification requires a scheme that circumvents the medical establishment either partially or altogether. So few people seek medical advice for the common cold, for example, that specially designed sample surveys of the population have been conducted to obtain an idea of the extent of the occurrence of colds. Facial tissue or cold nostrum sales would provide a considerably better estimate than would physician reports.

Also, physicians inevitably make errors, both of commission (overdiagnosis) and omission (underdiagnosis) in daily practice, despite their efforts to the contrary. Diagnostic misclassification results either from the intrinsic complexity or ambiguity of the symptoms and signs that the physician must consider to formulate a correct diagnosis, or from extraneous circumstances, such as the diagnostic acumen of the physician himself, his ability to communicate with the patient and vice versa, and access to necessary diagnostic aids. Either directly or indirectly, a physician's training, experience, and dedication to professional excellence will determine the extent to which he will err diagnostically; undoubtedly, the degree of diagnostic misclassification will vary from physician to physician.

There are a number of sources from which useful information can be procured when calculating disease rates in a population. These include official notifications (mandatory for many communicable diseases in most parts of the world), death registrations, reports of diagnostic laboratory tests, hospital and clinic records, health insurance claims, special disease registries (cancer, tuberculosis), and special population health surveys.

Many of the aforementioned sources provide data that leave something to be desired with respect to completeness. However, in most developed countries death registrations comprise virtually complete data sets relatable to discrete populations. Special registries, if well maintained, can also closely approximate death registrations with respect to completeness. The other information sources ordinarily provide only a partial enumeration and therefore reveal only the tip of the disease iceberg. This includes official notifications mandated by law. The information on diseases that is ascertained also is influenced by medical specialization. Pathologists' reports of autopsies will pertain only to the terminal portion of the disease spectrum; a family physician's contribution may include mild to moderately ill ambulatory patients for the most part, whereas the bulk of cases ascertained from an internist would more likely consist of atypical or severely ill cases.

Table 1 summarizes some of the factors that may contribute to incomplete case ascertainment of disease cases in a population.

Table 1

Sources and Causes of Errors in Ascertaining Disease Cases in Relation to the Disease Spectrum

	Cause of Error	
Source of Error	*Clinical Response Phase*	*Sequelae Phase*
1. Qualitative variability in disease expression (disease spectrum)	Asymptomatic cases; Atypical manifestations	Prolonged remission; Unexpected, sudden death
2. Patient behavior and access to medical care	Shame, fear, stoicism; Inability to communicate; Uncooperativeness; Prevarication (malingering or feigned illness); Lack of funds	Unauthorized hospital leaving; Change of residence; Change of physician; Abandoning medical service system; Mental disintegration
3. Physician behavior	Poor training; Carelessness; Diagnostic error; Nonnotification; Premature treatment	Failure to follow patient; Change of residence; Specialty restrictions
4. Medical and health service system	Laboratory error; Mislabeled reports; Lack of medical facilities	Lack of social services; Death from other causes; Death in another jurisdiction

The Rationale of Epidemiology

Epidemiological investigation is based on the premise that disease occurrence in populations is nonrandom. This negatively phrased declaration, "disease occurrence is nonrandom," becomes more explicit if couched positively, as Acheson has stated: " . . .all disease stems directly or indirectly from the patterns of men's lives . . ." "Patterns of men's lives" include genetic as well as environmental factors (nature-nurture interaction), which play a role in predisposing, producing, propagating, or perpetuating disease in populations.

Determinants of virtually any disease thus include factors related to the *agent, host,* and *environment.* Agents of disease include such things as dietary insufficiencies and excesses, chemical agents, allergens, physical agents, and infectious organisms. Host factors pertain to attributes of individuals that influence exposure to agents, and susceptibility to disease following exposure, such as genetic factors, age, sex, nutritional state, prior immunologic experience, and behavioral characteristics. Environmental factors include elements of the physical environment (such as climatic factors), aspects of the biologic environment (such as human population density and animals that may serve as reservoirs for human pathogens), and socioeconomic factors (such as certain occupations and various consequences of urbanization and poverty).

Factors in each of these three categories interact to produce disease. For example, the agent for smallpox is the variola virus; the environmental factor of crowding influences the probability that a well person will come in contact with a diseased person and thereby inhale the virus; and the vaccination status of the potential new host will determine whether he develops the disease following exposure. Coronary heart disease provides another example. Saturated fats and cholesterol may be considered agents; a high socioeconomic status is an environmental factor that increases the likelihood that persons will be exposed to large quantities of these agents; and a variety of complex genetic factors determine which individuals on a high-fat diet are most likely to develop the disease.

The various determinants of disease occurrence are termed *risk factors*. The aim of epidemiologic investigations of disease etiology is to identify and characterize such risk factors. This in turn provides the knowledge needed for the development and employment of preventive measures. Epidemiology is thus the basic science of preventive medicine.

Epidemiologic investigations are of three general types: *descriptive, analytic,* and *experimental*. Descriptive epidemiology utilizes information from population censuses for rate denominators. For numerator data, information available from such existing sources as death certificates, health department records of reportable diseases, and records of special registries is often utilized, or special surveys of existing medical records may be conducted. Incidence or mortality rates are then computed to provide a description of how the disease is distributed in the population with respect to time, place, and person. In this way, seasonal variation and long-term time trends in incidence are ascertained, areas with relatively high and low rates are identified, and individuals at increased risk are characterized by such characteristics as age, race, sex, and socioeconomic status. Such descriptions of the occurrence of a disease often provide hints as to what might be the cause of the disease in question, and provide ideas for more detailed analytic studies.

Analytic epidemiology pertains to the process of formulating and testing hypotheses as to the specific risk factors that might be determinants of a disease of interest. This usually implies conducting carefully designed studies in which data not available from existing records are collected and imaginatively analyzed.

Wade Hampton Frost, one of the early proponents of epidemiology in the United States wrote,

Epidemiology at any given time is something more than the total of its established facts. It includes their orderly arrangement into chains of inference that extend more-or-less beyond the bounds of direct observation. Chains such as these that are well and truly laid guide investigation to facts of the future; those that are ill laid fetter progress.*

---

*W.H. Frost, *An Introduction, Snow on Cholera* (London: The Commonwealth Fund, Oxford University Press 1936), page ix.

This quotation epitomizes the reasoning and reckoning that is epidemiology. When sufficient information about one or more risk factors is available from analytic studies, the stage is set for experimental studies involving intervention. Experimental epidemiology thus involves evaluating the effect that introducing, modifying, or reducing a risk factor has on the occurrence of a disease of interest. Water fluoridation and dental caries and vaccine field trials are examples.

Avenues of Epidemiologic Investigation

The following outline shows the avenues of investigation in humans that are used to attempt to identify environmental or genetic factors that may influence the occurrence of diseases in man.

Avenues of Investigation	*Information Obtained*
I. Clinical observations	Description of a case
II. Case studies (case series)	Description of a case series
III. Prevalence studies (cross-sectional)	Prevalence of disease
IV. Historically oriented studies	
A. Studies of incident events	
1. in general populations (descriptive studies)	Incidence or mortality rates
2. follow-up studies of specially selected groups (nonconcurrent prospective or historical cohort studies)	Incidence or mortality rates
B. Case-control studies (case-comparison or retrospective studies)	Prevalence of factor
V. Futuristically oriented studies	
A. Observational (concurrent prospective or futuristic cohort studies)	Incidence or mortality rates
B. Experimental (randomized trials or intervention studies)	Incidence or mortality rates

The first two avenues do not involve comparisons of rates and therefore are not epidemiologic approaches. Descriptive studies are included in avenue IV.A.1, and experimental studies are shown as avenue V.B. Avenues IV.A.2 through V.A generally denote analytic epidemiologic investigations, although some studies of incident events in general populations (IV.A.1) and some prevalence studies (III) may also be analytic.

A practicing physician may make a *clinical observation* that one or more of his patients developed a particular disease in an unusual situation (such as following treatment for a chronic medical condition, or while working in an unusual occupation). From this, he may hypothesize a causal relationship between some factor (such as a drug or chemical) and the disease. Such observations are frequently published in the medical literature as *case reports*. Although they obviously cannot provide firm evidence for a causal relationship, they may be of value in stimulating more formal investigations to confirm or refute suspected associations between various factors and disease.

Case studies are a logical extension of simple clinical observations. They are an attempt to collect and describe a *series* of cases of the same disease. Such series are often composed of all cases of the disease of interest that were seen by a particular physician, or in a particular clinic or hospital, or that occurred in a particular locality, during some specified period of time. Occasionally, information from case studies can provide strong evidence for an association between the disease and a suspected etiologic factor. This is particularly true when the disease is rare and the factor of interest is relatively new or uncommon. For example, a series of seven benign hepatomas (liver tumors) seen during a five-year period in Michigan was reported. All seven tumors occurred in women who had used oral contraceptives for from six months to five years. The rarity of the tumors, and the observation that they occurred only in women who had used oral contraceptives, rather strongly suggested to the investigators that oral contraceptives were somehow involved in the development of the tumors.

It must be emphasized, however, that this inference could not have been made if the investigators had been unable to assume reasonably that not all normal women of child-bearing age in Michigan had been users of oral contraceptives. If this assumption could not have been made, or if fewer than seven of the cases had been pill users, then the case series would not have been of value without a comparable series of women without liver tumors to which the case series could have been compared with respect to oral contraceptive use. Such studies, involving both a diseased and a nondiseased series, will be discussed in the section on case-control studies.

In *prevalence* (or *cross-sectional*) *studies*, the prevalence rates of a disease in defined groups or subsets of a population are compared. For example, the prevalence of carcinoma *in situ* of the uterine cervix was measured in two subsets of the population of women who attended a family planning clinic, and rates for women who used the diaphragm and those who used oral contraceptives were compared. Because rates were higher for the users of oral contraceptives, it was tentatively inferred either that these agents increase the risk of carcinoma *in situ* or, alternatively, that use of the diaphragm decreases the risk.

Historically oriented studies are of three types: descriptive, cohort, and case-control. Descriptive studies have been described. In *historical cohort studies*, also known as *nonconcurrent prospective studies*, groups of people who are characterizable at some time in the past by some factor of interest are identified from existing records and followed to determine what the incidence of one or more diseases or conditions has been in the interim. An example of this type of study is the measurement in recent years of the incidence of cardiovascular disease in men who graduated from a major U.S. university several decades ago. The incidence rates since graduation for those who did and did not participate in college athletics were compared to help determine whether physical exercise as a young man reduces the risk of cardiovascular disease.

Case-control studies (also known as *case-comparison* or *retrospective studies*), although also historically oriented, are distinctly different from historical cohort studies. Rather than starting with a group of essentially disease-free individuals and looking for subsequent disease, a group of already diseased persons (cases) is assembled, as are one or more groups of people largely without the disease in question (comparison groups or controls), and the proportion in each group with and without a past history of exposure to one or more factors of interest is ascertained. For example, to determine whether use of oral contraceptives (the factor) alters the risk of thromboembolism (the disease), a group of women with this disease and another group of women of the same age and race who were hospitalized for other reasons were studied. Because a higher proportion of women in the case group than in the comparison group gave a history of recent use of oral contraceptives, it was inferred that use of these hormonal preparations may increase the risk of thromboembolism.

Futuristic cohort studies are of two types: observational (also known as *concurrent prospective studies*) and experimental. In both types, groups of people are currently characterized by some factor of interest and followed forward in time to determine the future incidence of one or more diseases or conditions. Futuristic cohort studies of the observational type, like historical cohort studies, involve individuals who are not assigned to various groups by the investigator, but are merely observed as they already exist in such groups. Experimental studies, on the other hand, imply intervention by the investigator. A comparison of the future incidence of lung cancer in people who currently did and did not smoke cigarettes is an example of an observational cohort study. The investigators could not direct participants either to smoke or not to smoke, but merely observed those who were already smokers or nonsmokers. A vaccine field trial is an example of an experimental cohort study. Participants are randomly assigned to receive either vaccine or a placebo, and the subsequent incidence of disease in the two groups when compared can be used to determine the effectiveness of the vaccine.

Historically Oriented Investigations

Descriptive Studies

As we have seen, an epidemiologic investigation of a disease or condition usually begins by utilizing existing information to conduct a descriptive study. The arenas in which epidemiologists work may encompass hospitals, clinics, laboratories, and various community health agencies, all of which, as a matter of operational necessity, maintain extensive medical records containing raw material that may be suitable for epidemiologic investigations. The exploitation of existing available resources offers considerable savings in time, effort, and money over what would be expended if material were to be specially gathered.

Major disadvantages of utilizing such information collected for other purposes are: (1) lack of comparability of observations made by a variety of observers; (2) lack of uniformity in methods of recording observations; and often (3) critical omissions. Within the broad classification categories frequently employed in epidemiologic investigations, imperfect observations and records are often not of such poor quality as to render the study results without value so long as the quality of the data is not influenced by the fact of disease in case-control studies or by the presence of the factor of interest in cohort studies. A large proportion of missing information items, however, obviously severely compromises the usefulness of any material. The main limitation of descriptive studies is the small number and nonspecific nature of variables available.

Also, because historical material is usually incomplete for reasons discussed in the sections on the disease spectrum and the disease iceberg, values of rates should not be construed as exact, but rather as relative measures, suitable for perceiving trends but not representing the actual or true proportion of the population affected. If diagnostic and data collection practices do not remain stable over time, or differ from one area to another, incidence rates obtained from historical material cannot be depended upon for indicating actual trends or differences in risk in different areas. (A descriptive study is presented in problem 5.)

Nonconcurrent Prospective Studies

If the disease or condition of interest is to be studied in relation to variables other than those provided by routinely collected demographic or medical records (for example, smoking habits, occupational exposures, drug ingestion), an investigator can use either the prospective (cohort) or case-control avenues of investigation. If existing records of potential exposure to a factor of interest are available from special sources (such as industrial or school records), a formal *historical cohort study* can be mounted. This approach is limited, however, to those special situations in which the desired data on specific cohorts are already available. Epidemiologists frequently do not have the good fortune to find such data. In addition, such studies are expensive and administratively cumbersome because they usually require obtaining follow-up information on many thousands of individuals. In fact, the size of the cohorts that must be studied increases with the rarity of the condition of interest. Virtually all major chronic diseases of current importance in industrialized nations, for example, occur with such a low frequency as to make the application of this method to their study very expensive.

Case-Control Studies

For this reason, as well as others, the case-control study is the historical avenue more frequently used to provide additional epidemiologic information beyond what can be gleaned from existing demographic and medical records. The number of persons who must be studied by this method is dependent not on the frequency of the disease, but on the prevalence of the traits or factors of interest.

It will be recalled that the aim of the case-control approach is to compare the prevalence of traits or factors of interest in cases and in some comparison group. Ideally, the comparison group should provide the prevalence of the traits or factors in the population from which the cases derived. To obtain this prevalence in the population obviously requires some sort of population sample from which the desired proportions can be determined. By sampling, one can acquire a representative sample of the population at large to compare with an aggregate of cases stemming from the same population. Ideally, a sample of sufficient size would be selected at random in a deliberate and formal manner so that every person in the entire population would have an equal probability of being included in the sample. This would provide the most scientifically sound group for comparative purposes.

A properly drawn probability sample permits quantifying the degree to which chance alone might account for the results obtained. The confidence one can attach to the estimates obtained by sampling increases in proportion to the sample size.

Probability sampling may be feasible for ordinary descriptive purposes if the population is relatively small or is a closed one (institutions, for example) and if information is available on sampling units (individuals, households, tracts) that is necessary for the sampling process to be carried out. However, probability sampling of free-living populations often poses problems with respect to design and is expensive to carry out.

Instead of such probability samples, different sorts of *samples of convenience*, consisting of patients with diseases other than the one under investigation, neighbors, or other accessible individuals whose situation in life might be considered similar to the population at large, are often used to obtain at least a rough approximation of the prevalence of the factor of interest in the population for comparison with the prevalence in the patient group.

The credibility of the case-control avenue of investigation for eliciting associations of disease with specific factors hinges upon selection of a comparison group that can be taken as representative of the population from which the disease cases emanated. With samples of convenience, systematic bias in the selection of persons for comparison can occur. However, if a number of such crude samples, garnered by two or more investigators at different times and places, all reveal approximately the same association between trait and disease, then the findings can be viewed with considerable confidence.

Assembling a comparison group by the process of matching may eliminate obvious sources of systematic bias. Because age, sex, and ethnic group (or socioeconomic status, as one often predicts the other) may have a profound bearing on traits or factors of interest, these attributes are often used as matching variables. There is a practical limit to the number of variables that can be used for matching. If more than three or four are used, it becomes difficult, if not impossible, to successfully pair diseased individuals with those without disease unless an enormous number of persons comprise the pool from which the matched individuals can be drawn.

As an alternative to matching, and one that is preferred by an increasing number of investigators, information regarding suspected biasing factors is simply recorded for both case and comparison groups. The prevalence rates of the factor of interest, as well as the estimates of the degree of association between the factor of interest and the disease under study, can then be statistically adjusted to take into account the differences in composition of the two groups.

Prevalence Studies

We have seen that historically oriented investigations attempt to measure either the past mortality or incidence of disease (descriptive or historical cohort studies) or the prevalence of prior exposure to a factor (case-control study). In contrast to this historical approach, prevalence (or cross-sectional) studies seek to describe and compare the distribution of currently prevalent diseases or conditions in defined populations. This implies a two-step process: (1) defining the populations of interest, and (2) determining who in these populations currently has and does not have the disease or condition of interest.

The population may be a general one, such as all the people in a defined geographic areas, or a special one, such as all the people who, during a particular period of time, receive service from some organization (for example, a family planning clinic), work in some industry, or subscribe to a particular life style.

Once the populations of interest are defined, a population survey is conducted to detect those individuals who are and are not diseased. Testing a population, or even a sample fraction of a population, is ordinarily a task of such magnitude that a short-cut method for detecting the presence or absence of the condition becomes a necessity. Questionnaires or clinical tests of one sort or another (serological, biochemical, radiographical, cardiographical, cytological) are used for this purpose. Their use circumvents the labor of a complete medical examination for detecting disease. Such *screening tests*, however, may fail to find all cases of the disease, and they may result in well people erroneously being classified as having the diseases. These drawbacks are detailed in the section on sensitivity and specificity, but first we must consider the difference and relationship between reproducibility and accuracy.

Reproducibility and Accuracy

Test *reproducibility* (sometimes termed *reliability*) refers to the consistency with which a test yields the same result on the same specimen or subject by the same or different examiners on different occasions. In a laboratory setting, specimens can be divided into aliquots (portions) for repeat examination under circumstances that preclude the laboratorians' knowing the results of other runs until all have been completed (blind assessment). In a clinical or community setting, comparison of reports from two or more examiners concerning the presence or absence of specific facts elicited by medical history, physical examination, or special clinical tests (radiographs, electrocardiograph, blood pressure determinations), or concerning the manifest degree or extent of such facts, would provide evidence for or against the reliability of the particular observations.

Obviously, a test must be reproducible to be consistently accurate. However, a highly reproducible test is not necessarily an accurate one; a test can be consistently wrong.

The *accuracy* (also termed *validity*) of a test refers to its ability (including the ability of the person performing the test) to measure the actual or true state of the phenomenon being classified or quantified.

One type of inaccuracy is *digit preference*. For example, even individuals who are specially trained to measure blood pressure levels with an ordinary sphygmomanometer tend to read the gauge in such a manner that certain terminal digits appear with greater frequency than can be accounted for by chance. This is evidence of systematic bias (inaccuracy) in reading the scale. This phenomenon of terminal digit preference is demonstrated in the data in table 2, which are derived from a series of systolic and diastolic blood pressure determinations made on 79 separate individuals. The examiner (a scientist engaged in blood pressure research) recorded his results to the nearest even digit.

Table 2
Frequency of Terminal Digits Recorded for Blood Pressure
Determinations on 79 Individuals

Terminal Digit	Frequency (%)	
	Systolic	Diastolic
0	11	23
2	7	15
4	16	15
6	22	16
8	23	10

If one postulates that any one of the five terminal digits has the same probability of being recorded if the recorder were completely unbiased in his selection of the terminal digit (p = 0.2 or 20 percent) the expected frequency would be 15.8 for each one ($0.2 \times 79 = 15.8$). The table reveals that for systolic readings the digits 6 and 8 were recorded in excess of the expected frequency and for diastolic readings the terminal digit 0 was similarly distinguished. One is forced to conclude that despite the expertness of the recorder, the data reflect an element of observer subjectivity in reading the instrument gauge used in this test. Devices have been conceived (muddlers, averaging) in an attempt to minimize errors of this sort. If the test instrument is a questionnaire, validity (accuracy) may also be jeopardized by terminal digit preference in recalling dates, age, or other numerical facts.

The manner in which questions are phrased in a questionnaire (vague, leading, ambiguous, intimidating, insulting, ingratiating) may influence the accuracy of responses. Tests based on material of this sort are particularly prone to produce spurious results unless special steps are taken to establish the validity of an instrument of this type. Questions requiring recollection of events in the distant past obviously will yield less valid answers than those seeking recall of more recent ones—unless the respondent is elderly, in which case the opposite may be true. Questions addressed to the next of kin of individuals recently deceased may, in relation to certain sensitive topics (abuse of alcohol or other drugs for example), induce a "halo" response by the respondent such that he will reveal nothing derogatory (in his view, at least) concerning the deceased, even when it can be shown from other information that he has knowledge to the contrary.

The fact that a pathogenic organism is isolated from a patient may or may not be an accurate indication that the patient was infected by the organism. Colonization differs from infection. An accurate test for infection would entail showing evidence of host-agent interaction, such as immunological response or specific tissue changes.

A thermometer that is not correctly calibrated will surely produce inaccurate recordings of temperature.

These examples indicate that the accuracy of a test can be influenced by factors related to the observer, the study subject, or the instruments employed.

In prevalence studies (population surveys, cross-sectional surveys), a test is generally used to classify persons as either with or without some disease, trait, or condition. There are two measures of how precisely any specific test does so—sensitivity and specificity. These two very important epidemiologic concepts are discussed in the following section.

Sensitivity and Specifity

Sensitivity and *specificity* are complementary measures of the validity of a test, procedure, or diagnostic criterion. Sensitivity indicates the proportion (or percentage) of diseased individuals that will be identified as diseased by the test, and specificity indicates the proportion of nondiseased individuals that will be designated disease-free by the test.

These two concepts are illustrated in tables 3 and 4. Individuals with the disease in question who have a positive test result are true positives, and those with the disease who have a negative test result are false negatives. Similarly, persons without the disease who have a negative test result are true negatives, and those without the disease who have a positive test result are false positives.

Table 3
Contingencies of Testing for Disease

Groups Tested	Test Results		Totals
	Positive	Negative	
Disease	True positives	False negatives	Total diseased
Nondisease	False positives	True negatives	Total nondiseased

Sensitivity = true positives/total diseased; Specificity = true negatives/total nondiseased

Table 4
Contingencies of Testing for Disease: Numerical Example

Groups Tested	Test Results		Totals
	Positive	Negative	
Disease	180	30	210
Nondisease	27	300	327

Sensitivity = 180/210 × 100 = 85.7%; Specificity = 300/327 × 100 = 91.7%

Sensitivity is thus the proportion of diseased persons who are true positives, and specificity is the proportion of nondiseased persons who are true negatives.

In clinical terms, the sensitivity of a symptom, sign, or diagnostic test is the proportion of diseased individuals that will have the symptom, exhibit the sign, or have an abnormal test result.

Traditionally, information on signs and symptoms originates from a review of hospital charts or clinic records of patients with a certain diagnosis, with the reviewer noting the recorded presence or absence of certain symptoms or signs for each patient. Results of such analysis ordinarily appear as a list of symptoms and signs ranked according to the relative frequency (usually expressed in percentage) with which they were recorded. Although such results are, in fact, measures of sensitivity, it has not been customary to use the term in connection with clinical material so much as with information derived from laboratory tests or specialized diagnostic procedures.

In clinical terms, the specificity of a symptom, sign, or diagnostic test is a measure of its uniqueness in relation to the disease in question. If it is highly specific, it is *pathognomonic* for the disease, which is to say that few or no other conditions are characterized by the same symptom, sign, or test result.

If the sensitivity of a test were 100 percent, there would be no false negatives, and if the specificity were 100 percent, there would be no false positives. This ideal situation is never achieved because of factors already mentioned in connection with the diagnostic process, test accuracy, and reproducibility, as well as other factors that mar perfection, including such human foibles as carelessness, prevarication, misunderstanding, uncooperativeness, and "a bad day."

Murphy's Law ("if something can go wrong, it will") virtually guarantees that although a value of 100 percent may be theoretically possible, such a value has an exceedingly low probability of happening in practice and, if encountered, should be viewed with skepticism. Corrigan's Corollary ("Murphy is an incorrigible optimist") accentuates the point.

Obviously, in screening a population for case-finding purposes, one would wish for a test that was both highly sensitive and highly specific, so that misclassification of both cases and noncases would be minimal. Some interesting and sometimes disastrous consequences attend the application of disease-screening tests to populations, as the next section will reveal.

Sensitivity, Specificity, and Disease Prevalence

Suppose that on review of the pertinent literature one learns that a test for a particular disease rated high in terms of both sensitivity (95 percent) and specificity (97 percent). Assuming that the test involved little if any discomfort to the person submitting to it (high acceptability), it would seem to be a feasible means for screening a population to establish the prevalence rate of the disease. Because one would expect some false positives (specificity 97 percent, not 100 percent), each positive reactor would be a candidate for referral for formal medical consultation to establish or disestablish the diagnosis.

Under these circumstances, if the actual prevalence rate of the disease in a population of 100,000 persons to be screened equaled 5 per 1,000, there would be 500 cases that could be detected. With a sensitivity of 95 percent, the test could be expected to identify 475 of these correctly ($0.95 \times 500 = 475$) and would miss 25 ($0.05 \times 500 = 25$). With a specificity of 97 percent, the test would correctly classify 96,515 as well ($99,500 \times 0.97 = 96,515$), but 2,985 ($99,500 \times 0.03 = 2,985$) would be wrongly categorized as diseased (false positives). The sum of the positive test reactors composed of the 475 true positives and the 2,985 false positives, totaling 3,460, would comprise the numerator of a prevalence rate based on the application of this test. Divided by the total number tested (100,000), the estimated rate would equal 34.6 per 1,000, as opposed to the true prevalence rate of 5 per 1,000—a miss of the mark by a factor of almost 7.

The villain here is the large number of noncases that were wrongly classified as diseased, despite a high test specificity. If each of the 3,460 persons with a positive test result were to be referred to a physician to rule in or rule out the presence of disease, the cost in time, money, effort, and patience of the doctors involved could be staggering, and many well persons would have been falsely alarmed.

Many well-intentioned community efforts have foundered and embarrassed their instigators, who had not considered the arithmetic consequences of their good intentions. The critical ingredient with respect to population screening is the true disease prevalence rate. Table 5 demonstrates the effect of an increasing true prevalence rate on the rate estimated from a test with a sensitivity of 95 percent and a specificity of 97 percent in a population of 100,000.

This table indicates that community-wide screening programs will generate major errors in identifying those with and without disease. For example, with a true prevalence of 25, the estimated prevalence was 53 (more than twice the

Table 5

Consequence of Estimating Prevalence Using a Test Instrument with 95% Sensitivity and 97% Specificity

True Prevalence Rate/1,000	Number of True Positives	Number of False Positives	Estimated Prevalence Rate/1,000	Number of False Negatives
5	475	2,985	34.6	25
25	2,375	2,925	53.0	125
125	11,875	2,625	145.2	625
625	59,375	1,125	605.9	3,125

real value). The true prevalence figure of 125 per 1,000 (12.5 percent) was approximated fairly closely by the estimate based on the test, but 2,625 well people were erroneously designated as being diseased, and 625 true cases were missed. At a true prevalence of 625 per 1,000 (over 50 percent), the test under-estimates the prevalence of the disease. The lesson to be learned from this analysis is that even a test with high sensitivity and specificity may not yield accurate results unless its use is restricted to relatively small population subsets in which the prevalence is suspected as being substantial. Examples of this are screening contacts of typhoid fever cases for evidence of infection, and screen-ing female relatives of a person with hemophilia to identify carriers. Diagnostic classification based on individuals who react positively to two or more tests rather than just one offers a practical solution to the problem, but at increased cost. (Problem 6 deals with some practical aspects of sensitivity and specificity.)

Variable-Specific Rates and Rate Adjustment

Because age plays a cardinal role in disease determination, arranging disease rates by successive age groups is a standard practice in epidemiologic investiga-tion. The pattern of distribution by age for a number of diseases is highly specific; in fact, some medical specialties, such as pediatrics and geriatrics, evolved because of the relationship of age with certain kinds of disease that require special skills for their diagnosis and treatment. Death rates by age groups provide an instructive example of a pattern common throughout the world.

Figure 8 contrasts the overall mortality experience in 1970 of a largely rural population living in a tropical environment (West Malaysia), numbering 4,648,377 according to a census in August 26, 1970, with a population of 3,409,169 persons on April 1, 1970, residing in the temperate climate of Wash-ington State in a predominantly industrialized society. The graph illustrates a phenomenon that has come to be accepted as a commonplace difference between developed and developing countries, largely attributable to standard-of-living disparities. The greatest proportional differences appear in the younger age groups; after the age of 35, these differences tend to diminish progressively with advancing years.

Note that the ordinate (vertical axis) of the graph is scaled logarithmically. This scale serves two purposes. First, it enables one to plot numbers that differ greatly in order of magnitude on conventional-sized paper, while at the same time illuminating trends in the small-number end of the range, which would be obscured by their proximity to the abscissa (horizontal axis) on an arithmetic scale. The rates plotted on the graph ranged from 0.4 to 70.1—over a hundred-fold difference in magnitude. Second, a logarithmic scale has the mathematical property of depicting differences proportionately rather than in absolute terms.

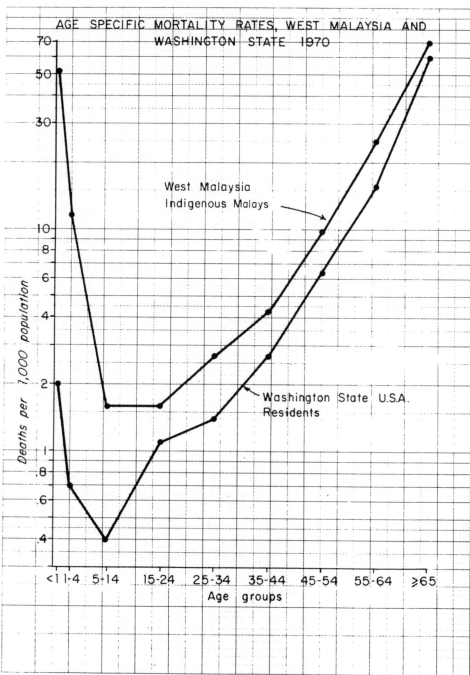

Figure 8. Age-Specific Mortality, West Malaysia and Washington State, 1970

By examining the scale on the graph, one can verify that the vertical distance from 0.3 to 0.6 is the same as that from 3.0 to 6.0 and, in turn, the same as that from 30.0 to 60.0—a doubling in each instance. Thus, the difference in rates between Malays and Washingtonians aged 25 to 34 years is proportionately greater than that at ages 45 to 54, for example. The absolute differences can be obtained by subtracting the appropriate scale values. One disadvantage of a semilogarithmic graph is that low absolute values appear relatively large when, in fact, they are small.

In addition to age, sex plays a crucial role with respect to disease predisposition and also with respect to survival. The specialties of obstetrics and gynecology developed in response to unique problems of diagnosis and management of disorders peculiar to the female sex. Figure 9 presents the same material as Figure 8, but it has been subdivided by sex as well as age. From this plot the discrepancy between Washington male and female rates stands in marked contrast to the Malay pattern; for every age group the rate for Washington males exceeds that for females by a good margin, whereas the rate for Malay females equals or exceeds that for males in the groups 15 to 24, 25 to 34, and 35 to 44, the childbearing years. This observation undoubtedly reflects health disadvantages that stem from social, cultural, economic, and other factors.

A problem arises in comparing rates for two populations that differ in composition with respect to age, sex, and any other factor that can influence disease patterns. Obviously, a population that has a larger proportion of people in a particular subset that has a high disease rate will have a higher overall disease rate by virtue of this disproportion. Examination of rates specific for subsets that might produce a distortion of the overall rates would readily reveal that the overall rates should not be compared unless some correction is made for the difference in population composition. The statistical technique for correcting confounding variables is termed *rate adjustment* or *rate standardization.*

The process of adjusting or standardizing a crude or overall disease rate for a factor involves the use of rates specific for the factor. For example, if the factor were age, then rates specific for each age group in the population selected for rate adjustment would be used. A separate population, subdivided into corresponding age groups, is used as a standard of reference. Multiplying each age-specific rate from the population selected for rate adjustment by the number of persons in the corresponding age group in the standard population yields the number of disease cases that would be expected to occur in the standard population if the standard population had an age-specific disease rate experience identical to that of the population selected for rate adjustment. The sum of the expected number of disease cases from each age group constitutes the numerator of the adjusted or standardized rates. The sum of all the individuals in each age group of the standard population provides the denominator for the adjusted rate. Crude rates for one or several populations can be adjusted against the same standard population and then compared one with the other on the premise that

39

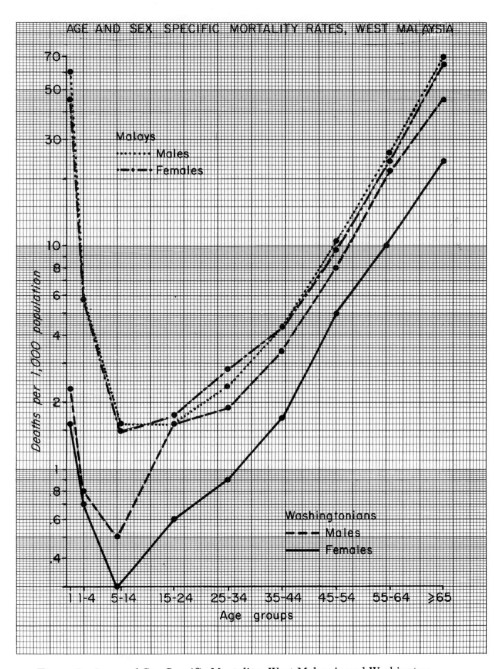

Figure 9. Age- and Sex-Specific Mortality, West Malaysia and Washington
State, 1970

any differences noted can be explained not by differences in the age composition of the populations but by some factor other than age, because the age factor has been taken into account.

The rates obtained by this means (the so-called direct method for standardization) will be fictitious in the sense that their magnitude will depend upon the population selected as the standard. Of interest is not the magnitude of the adjusted rate but whether one adjusted rate is larger or smaller compared with the other. The relationship of one rate to the other after adjustment for one or more factors can be assumed to be the effect of factors other than those used for standardization. Table 6 shows the steps for computation of adjusted rates using hypothetical data chosen so as to simplify the arithmetic and clarify the principles involved. In this example, sex rather than age is the factor for which an adjustment is made, and the sum of populations A and B is arbitrarily used as the standard population.

After adjustment, the difference in rates between A and B is slightly greater than that obtained by comparison of the crude rates. (Problem 7 deals with rate adjustment utilizing the data depicted in Figures 8 and 9.

Table 6
Standardization of Rates: Example of the Direct Method

		Population Groups to be Compared	
Computation Sequence		*A*	*B*
Census (total population)		100	100
Disease cases		13	7
Crude rate (%)		13.0	7.0
Census (male)		30	50
Cases (male)		8	4
Rate for males (%)		26.6	8.0
Census (female)		70	50
Cases (female)		5	3
Rate for females (%)		7.1	6.0
Standard population			
Males (population $A + B$)		80	
Females (population $A + B$)		120	
Calculated	Males	$0.226 \times 80 = 21.3$	$0.080 \times 80 = 6.4$
expected number	Females	$0.071 \times 120 = 8.5$	$0.060 \times 120 = 7.2$
of cases in standard			
population	Total	29.8	13.6
Total standard population		200	
Sex-adjusted rate (%)		$\dfrac{29.8}{200} = 14.9$	$\dfrac{13.6}{200} = 6.8$

Cohort Analysis

Age-specific incidence or mortality rates for successive time periods in a single geographic area can be used to estimate the risk of disease in individual *age cohorts* (groups of people born during the same time period). The technique used is termed *cohort analysis*. Table 7 provides data to illustrate how this analysis is performed. Mortality from cancer of the lung and bronchus in succeeding generations of U.S. males serves as an example.

Because virtually all lung and bronchus cancer victims die within a few years following onset and because the diagnostic criteria have not changed appreciably over the span of the 30 years depicted in the table, these mortality rates may be construed as adequately reflecting incidence rates for the various age groups at successive ten-year intervals. The table can be viewed in three ways:

1. *Down the columns.* If these rates were plotted on a graph, column by column, the series of curves generated would show the relationship of disease rates to age for each of the succession of calendar decades.

2. *Across the rows.* Plotting the rates across each row generates a series of curves that shows the change in rates with calendar time for each of the age groups.

3. *Diagonally from the left downward to the right.* This technique defines the experience of people born during successive ten-year periods with respect to their risk of dying from cancer of the lung and bronchus as they become older. For example, those people born between 1920 and 1929 comprise the 10 to 19 age group in 1940, with a rate of 0.15 per 100,000; by 1950 they constituted the 20 to 29 age group, whose rate was 0.6 per 100,000. By 1960 their rate increased to 4.0.

Each successive cohort represents males who were, on the average, ten years older than the preceding group. Plotting each of the diagonals will generate curves for the various cohorts and reflect the influence of both age and factors related to calendar time. Each successive cohort can be seen to have

Table 7
Mortality Rates per 100,000 Due to Cancer of the Lung and Bronchus for U.S. Males by Age and for Selected Years from 1930 to 1960

Age Groups	1930	1940	1950	1960
0–9	0	0	0	0
10–19	0.12	0.15	0.2	0.3
20–29	0.3	0.4	0.6	0.8
30–39	1.2	2.0	2.5	4.0
40–49	4.0	10.0	15.0	25.0
50–59	10.0	30.0	60.0	95.0
60–69	16.0	41.0	90.0	170.0
70–79	14.0	38.0	85.0	180.0
80–89	7.5	25.0	65.0	130.0

experienced a higher rate of lung and bronchus cancer than the preceding cohort. This has been attributed to greater use of cigarettes by succeeding cohorts. Such a phenomenon is termed *cohort effect*.

The word *cohort* derives from the Latin, which originally signified a military unit of the Roman legions, similar to a modern military company, that was intended to serve as a single tactical force that was kept intact. Cohorts need not be defined for epidemiological purposes only with respect to time of birth but can be assembled on the basis of any attribute that distinguishes a subset of the population. Cohorts of persons emigrating from a certain place at successive time intervals or persons beginning their lifelong occupation during consecutive periods could be similarly studied.

Concurrent Prospective Studies

The first step in planning a concurrent prospective investigation is the recruitment of contemporary cohorts of individuals, one cohort being distinguishable from one or more others on the basis of the presence, absence, or difference in degree of one or more specific factors suspected of altering the probability of contracting the disease in question. Cohorts may consist of entire populations, selected population subsets, or samples of a population.

Ideally, there should be assurance that members of cohort groups are free of the disease to be investigated at the time the cohorts are assembled, so that subsequent disease incidence can be logically related to factors under study without being confounded by preexisting but unidentified disease. Furthermore, the groups should be similar in composition with respect to factors not under study that are related to the disease of interest. If not, salient differences with respect to these factors should be recorded so that appropriate adjustments can be made in the analysis of the results. Provision must be made for surveillance of each cohort to detect incident cases. The length of the surveillance period will depend upon the anticipated incidence rate (estimated from previous historically oriented investigation) and the size of the cohorts being monitored.

The process of studying the natural history of a disease by observing its course in various categories of patients is also a cohort study.

The major advantage of prospective avenues of investigation is that the disease rates obtained measure risk of disease directly with respect to factors identified before the disease event occurred. An additional advantage of concurrent prospective studies over nonconcurrent prospective studies is that investigators performing the former can study a disease of interest in relation to any variable they are able to measure in the study subjects; they are not restricted to consideration of variables on which data from existing sources are already available.

The major disadvantage of this method is largely one of expense; the cost in effort, time, and money has to be considered and adjudicated in the light of the benefits expected. The size of the cohorts that must be studied increases with the rarity of the disease under investigation. For this reason, the concurrent prospective avenue of investigation is usually reserved for special situations that warrant direct estimates of risk. For example, suppose that a case-control investigation indicates a strong statistical association between a disease and a particular factor. This sort of information is inadequate for advising someone with the factor what the probability of his developing the disease in the future might be. Only a prospective investigation can provide this kind of information.

Comparing Rates

We stated earlier in this text that epidemiologic fundamentals would be presented in the context of their pertinence to disease rates: their composition, the process of acquiring their components, and their interpretation. The section entitled "The Rationale of Epidemiology" dealt with the matter of disease-rate interpretation in general terms with respect to the ultimate goals of epidemiologic investigation but not with respect to specific techniques that facilitate the translation of numbers into meaningful facts.

Except for indicating magnitude (large, infinitesimal, or somewhere in between), a single disease rate, by itself, is virtually devoid of meaning; rates take on epidemiological significance primarily by appropriate comparisons with other rates. The simplest situation would entail the comparison of two rates by noting that one was larger or smaller than the other or that the two were, for practical purposes, identical. This observation may or may not convey information that is useful for a particular epidemiological purpose.

It is sometimes useful to compare rates according to the extent by which they differ in magnitude by measuring the difference. For example, in investigating outbreaks of suspected food-borne disease, one interrogates each person who may have been exposed to the disease agent (by virtue of having been present at a given meal) concerning suspected food items he or she ate or did not eat: such a history is obtained for both those who became ill and those who did not. For such information, incidence rates (or attack rates) can be calculated for those who ate and those who did not eat each food item. If the list of items exceeds four or five in number, inspecting the rate differences instead of rate pairs facilitates the interpretation. Table 8 illustrates this situation.

One can readily perceive from the right-hand column of this table that the attack rate difference between those eating and not eating turkey exceeds the differences for any other food items by a considerable margin and therefore points to turkey as the most likely vehicle of infection in this outbreak. Rate

Table 8
Food-Associated Epidemic: Analysis of Attack Rates by Food Items

Food Item	Attack Rates (%)		Attack Rate Difference
	Those Eating	Those Not Eating	
Fruit cocktail	81	55	26
Milk	81	75	6
Roll	80	68	12
Turkey	81	2	79
Gravy	83	54	29
Dressing	81	50	31
Potatoes	79	50	29
Peas	87	60	27
Apple cobbler	81	67	14
Coffee	78	75	3

differences are sometimes referred to as *attributable rates* on the premise that, other factors being equal, the difference in rate pairs can be attributed to the factor being investigated.

Ratios of rates (dividing one rate of a pair by the other) are termed *relative rates* because the ratio expresses the magnitude of one rate relative to that of the other. This expedient enables one to say that one rate is so many times larger than another rate or that one rate exceeds another by a factor of so much. In the attack-rate-by-food-item analysis, the relative rate for the food item, turkey, equals 40.5 (81/2), which would be interpreted as an indication that the attack rate for those eating turkey was over 40 times greater than for those not eating this food item. The relative attack rate for dressing, the item with the second highest attributable rate, equals 1.6 (81/50), which stands in marked contrast to the value of 40.5 for turkey.

Relative rates dramatize rate relationships more than do attributable rates but at the same time, because they are ratios and therefore unitless, they give no indication of the actual rate values with which one is dealing. For example, a relative rate of 10 could be derived from a comparison of a rate of 100 per 1,000 population with a rate of 10 per 1,000 population or from a comparison of rates of 10 per 100,000 and 1 per 100,000.

Unfortunately, the terms *attributable rate* and *relative rate* often engender more confusion than erudition; they are mentioned here only because they have been and still are used by some investigators. The terms *rate difference* and *rate ratio* would seem preferable, if for no other reason than to simplify the semantics and thereby enhance communication.

If more than two rates are to be compared, a common practice is to rank them in order of magnitude from lowest to highest, or vice versa, in order to see if an epidemiologically meaningful pattern can be perceived. One looks for uniform gradients of rate values if the factor for which the rate has been calculated would logically be expected to produce a trend up or down consonant with a concomitant change in the factor. For example, if one were to calculate disease rates for population groups whose life circumstance or style could expose them differently to an agent suspected of producing the disease, then the rates should be lowest for those suspected of having the least exposure, higher for those with more exposure, and highest for those most exposed. Such an observation would suggest a *dose response*, and would be strong evidence that the suggested agent was responsible for producing the disease.

Imputing Risk and Associations from Disease Rates

Because incidence rates indicate the proportion of a population affected with a particular disease or condition during a defined period of time, they may be construed, with reservation, as measures of *risk*. That is, they indicate the chance of an individual in the population being affected. The process of imputing risk from disease rates differs somewhat from formal probability estimation based on the laws of probability. The first law of probability states that the probability of an event cannot be less than zero nor greater than one. Under certain circumstances encountered in epidemiologic investigation, the numerator figure may be larger than the denominator, so that the rate for the period specified exceeds one, that is, is greater than 100 percent. Obviously, this indicates that some individuals in the population were affected more than once during the period, with either recurrences or relapses. Sexually exuberant ships' crews have been reported to have had venereal disease rates (gonorrhea) in excess of 100 percent during a specified time interval (shore leave), for example. It is likely that in some populations of children, the annual incidence of the common cold might be in the neighborhood of 200 percent or 300 percent. For the most part, however, the numerators of disease rates are but a small part of their denominators and therefore can be taken to represent observed probabilities from which risk can be inferred.

The ratio of two incidence rates, known as the *risk ratio*, or *relative risk*, is a *measure of association* commonly used by epidemiologists. For example, if the incidence rates of lung cancer among male smokers and nonsmokers are found to be 85.2 and 14.7 per 100,000 men per year, respectively, then these represent the corresponding risks to smokers and nonsmokers. The ratio of these two rates is 85.2 ÷ 14.7 = 5.8. This is a measure of the association between smoking and lung cancer, and it means that (in this example), the incidence of lung cancer is 5.8 times greater for smokers than for nonsmokers. It should be noted that although underascertainment of cases will result in spuriously low measures of incidence (and hence of risk), the relative risk is unaffected by this deficiency unless the degree of underassessment is different for smokers and nonsmokers.

As was indicated in the section on avenues of investigation, incidence rates are computed from any type of cohort study. It follows, then, that relative risks can be directly computed from the results of any such investigation. On the other hand, incidence rates are not obtained from prevalence or case-control studies. Even so, relative risks can be estimated from such investigations and used as measures of association.

In prevalence studies, the ratio of two prevalence rates is used as the estimate of the relative risk. The validity of the results of any prevalence study thus depends on the degree to which the ratio of prevalence rates reflects what would have been observed if the ratio of incidence rates could have been ascertained. This will vary with the circumstances of each investigation.

In case-control studies, the estimate of the relative risk is less intuitive than in cross-sectional investigations. It can be calculated, however. The results of any case-control study, which is conducted to measure the association between some disease and some putative causative factor, can be displayed in a two-by-two table, as follows:

Factor	Cases	Controls
Yes	a	b
No	c	d
Total	$m = a + c$	$n = b + d$

Note that m cases are studied, of which a are found to have been exposed to the factor and c of which have not. Similarly, n individuals have been assembled as a comparison group, b of whom were found to have been exposed and d of whom were not. The relative risk, RR, is estimated by the *cross products ratio,* which is given by the following formula:

$$RR = \frac{ad}{bc}$$

When cases and controls are matched to each other on a one-to-one basis, a different formula is often used to give a more precise estimate of the relative risk, although results seldom differ appreciably from those obtained using the formula above. (Problems 8 and 9 deal with prospective and case-control studies, respectively.)

In the course of an epidemiologic investigation of a disease or condition, one often seeks to identify as many variables (factors, attributes) as possible that are associated with the disease in question. This procedure often generates a veritable web of associations. The phrase web of associations implies that the observed associations (relative risks) will be confounded to a greater or lesser extent by the interrelationship between the various factors. Sophisticated statistical techniques have been developed to measure the true association between specific factors and a disease, taking into account such interrelationships between variables. From the matrix of relative risks one thereby seeks to identify factors that may actually be responsible for disease occurrence beyond what might be expected by chance alone.

A simple statistical association between a factor and a disease is not the only evidence that the epidemiologist uses to determine whether the association is a causal one. He also reviews the literature to determine whether there has been *replication* of his findings by other investigators. In addition, he considers the *strength of the association*; a very strong association is less likely to be due to factors other than a cause-effect relationship than a weak one. *Consistency of results* also favors a causal interpretation; the epidemiologist therefore analyzes subsets of his data to determine whether the association is consistently present in such subgroups as the two sexes, various age groups, and different races. He also looks for evidence of a *dose response*, which is a strong indicator of cause; and he considers whether the association is *biologically plausible* in light of what is known of the biological activity of the factor and the pathogenesis of the disease in humans and other animal species.

Another piece of evidence for causation is evidence that cessation of exposure reduces the risk of disease. Such evidence is sometimes available from analytic studies. It is also sometimes obtained from experimental studies, an avenue of investigation that is also used to test the efficacy of various preventive and curative measures.

Experimental Studies

Two features of experimental studies (or trials) distinguish them from concurrent prospective studies. These are *allocation* of study subjects by the investigators into two or more groups (often called *treatment groups* even though one group may serve as a control group), and *intervention*. Allocation is usually accomplished by a process of *randomization*, in which chance alone determines to which treatment group each person is assigned. The type of intervention (or lack of it) is, of course, what distinguishes the various treatment groups. The various groups are then prospectively observed, and incidence rates of disease (or other measures of outcome) in the various groups are compared.

Investigators intent upon gaining knowledge may seriously prejudice the results of a trial by their overenthusiastic expectations or fixed commitment to a preconceived result. Observer bias goes hand-in-glove with participant bias. Subjects of investigation typically tend to try to oblige the investigator by reporting what they think he wants them to report. Such mutual self-delusion can wreak havoc with objective appraisal of a trial outcome. To eliminate these sources of error, *double-blind* techniques are employed whenever possible. This term refers to the fact that neither the subjects nor the investigators who are treating or observing them have knowledge of what treatment group any subject is in. This is accomplished by administering indistinguishable treatments to each subject. Controls may receive an inert substance, termed a *placebo*, that resembles the substance being tested in as many respects as practical (appearance, taste, smell, and so forth).

Experimental studies conducted to determine whether a particular factor is a cause of a disease usually involve eliminating the suspected factor from one study group and not the other. An example of this is a current collaborative study in which healthy individuals at high risk of myocardial infarctions were randomly assigned either to a control group that received only routine medical care as needed, or to an experimental group that received a number of inducements to, among other things, reduce their intake of saturated fatty acids and cholesterol. The incidence of myocardial infarction in both groups will be compared to determine whether the intervention reduced the risk of disease. If so, this would constitute strong evidence that dietary fats are a cause of myocardial infarctions, and it would demonstrate that this disease can be partly prevented by dietary modification. Because of the logistics involved, this study obviously cannot be double-blind.

Experimental principles apply to the evaluation of other preventive measures, such as vaccines, and to the evaluation of therapeutic measures, such as new drugs (by means of clinical trials). These studies are usually performed using double-blind techniques.

When two treatment groups are compared to evaluate a preventive measure, the incidence rate for each may be used to calculate the *protection rate* (synonymous with effectiveness or efficacy rate). If the incidence rate for the cohort receiving the prophylactic were 2.2 per 100 and for the cohort receiving the placebo 15.9 per 100, the protection rate would be the difference (attributed to the prophylactic effect) expressed as a percentage of the rate for the cohort that was not protected. Thus:

$$\text{Protection rate (\%)} = \frac{\text{Incidence rate unprotected} - \text{Incidence rate protected}}{\text{Incidence rate unprotected}} \times 100$$

or

$$1 - \frac{\text{Incidence rate protected}}{\text{Incidence rate unprotected}} \times 100$$

From the figures cited:

$$1 - 2.2/15.9 \times 100 = 86\%$$

The protection rate may be interpreted as expressing the number of people protected by the prophylactic for every 100 people who receive it. The protection rate, which summarizes two rates in a single figure, is especially useful for comparing the results of several trials of the same prophylactic or individual trials of different prophylactics being evaluated for the prevention of a single disease. (Problem 10 deals with an intervention study to test the effect of vitamin C as a preventive of respiratory illness. Problem 11 provides a review of many of the important epidemiologic avenues of investigation.)

The Rubella Story

The chronicle of investigation of the association between rubella (German measles, three-day measles) in pregnant women and the occurrence of congenital defects in their babies aptly recapitulates many of the concepts and principles described in the foregoing material.

The clinical observations of an Australian ophthalmologist, N. McAlister Gregg,* prompted a series of subsequent investigations that did not cease until 30 years later when, finally, sufficient facts were in hand to put the original discovery into proper scientific perspective.

Between 1939 and 1941 an extensive epidemic of German measles (rubella) occurred in Australia, involving many adults as well as children. In retrospect, it was assumed that the physical isolation of Australia from the rest of the world, and in addition the relative isolation of communities within the country itself, had permitted the accumulation of a large number of susceptible young adults as well as children. It could not be established whether rubella had been endemic in Australia prior to the epidemic or was periodically reintroduced by visitors. However, it was ascertained that rubella incidence had been low since the mid 1920s, which would account for susceptibility of many young adults in the 1939–1940 epidemic. This epidemic was assumed to have been triggered by the military mobilization of World War II.

In the course of his practice, Gregg began to recognize infants with cataracts (opacity of the lens of the eye) that were clinically and pathologically different from cataracts he had been trained to diagnose. He noted, also, that many of the affected babies were inordinately small, difficult to feed, and had evidences of congenital heart disease. Gregg noted that the mothers of these infants had become pregnant coincidently with the peak of the rubella epidemic. Realizing that the critical period of embryonic eye development occurs during the first few weeks of fetal life, he queried the mothers of babies with the unusual cataracts concerning the occurrence of rubella during their pregnancies. Their responses prompted him to solicit additional information from his colleagues practicing in different parts of Australia. Some of his findings are summarized in Table 9.

---

*N. McAlister Gregg, "Congenital Cataract Following German Measles in the Mother." *Trans. Ophthal. Soc. Austral.* 3:35–36 (1941).

Table 9
The Association of Congenital Cataracts and Rubella during Pregnancy

Source of Cases	Number with Congenital Cataracts	Number with History of Rubella during Pregnancy
Gregg	13	12
Other ophthalmologists	65	56
Total	78	68

Gregg discovered that the reported rubella illness almost always occurred during the first two months of pregnancy, and he postulated that the unusual cataracts, and concomitant heart disease as well, may have been produced by the rubella infection during the early months of intrauterine life, when the fetal tissues were undergoing critical phases of development.

Impressive as the data are ($68/78 \times 100 = 87$ percent of cases with maternal rubella history), some important questions must be answered before a cause and effect relationship can be inferred. The 87 percent figure represents the proportion with cataracts who also had been exposed to rubella virus *in utero*. Without this prevalence rate among women who delivered normal babies at about the same time, the association between cataract and rubella during pregnancy cannot definitely be determined, although the rate of 87 percent was so high as to cause suspicion.

Gregg's publication excited the interest of the scientific community the world over; here was an opportunity to learn about a congenital disease problem that, unlike so many other congenitally acquired diseases, might be found amenable to some sort of preventive intervention. A number of historically oriented epidemiological and clinical investigations conducted during the ensuing years not only confirmed the association that Gregg suspected but also revealed that the spectrum of disease was considerably broader than originally perceived. In addition to cataract, heart defects, and growth retardation, all of which might be perceptible at the time of birth or soon afterward, it became obvious that defects that became clinically detectable only later in life were also related. Deafness and mental retardation emerged as additional major manifestations; enlargement of the spleen (splenomegally) and liver (hepatomegally) and a peculiar radiographic appearance of the leg bones, resembling a celery stalk, became recognized as components of the congenital rubella syndrome. In time, still another variant of disease expression became recognized; some affected children were born with a florid rubella rash and were found to be shedding rubella virus, indicating persisting activity of the infection months after the process began—a phenomenon at variance with the usual pattern of viral replication and proliferation, which generally lasts only a matter of days.

Eventually, several futuristically oriented epidemiological investigations were undertaken in response to the obvious necessity for assessing directly the risk of the serious consequences of congenital rubella that a woman who acquired rubella infection during pregnancy might expect. Such studies were initiated in Sweden, Great Britain, Australia, and the United States at about the same time; the following account details the method and results of a prospective investigation carried out in New York City which was published in 1971* (30 years after Gregg's paper).

The study design provided for longitudinal investigation of all cases of rubella reported by physicians in New York City involving females of child-bearing age during the period 1957 through 1964. Within 48 hours of notification, the woman who was reported to have rubella was examined in her home by a health department epidemiologist for clinical evidence of the disease, in order to corroborate the diagnosis, and was interrogated concerning her marital status and menstrual history. Those deemed to have the disease and to have been pregnant at its onset were enrolled in the study and observed through the balance of their pregnancy, and their liveborn offspring were examined repeatedly by pediatricians for growth and psychomotor defects, hearing loss, and cardiac abnormalities up to the age of five years—an impressive undertaking.

A comparison group of unaffected mothers and their offspring were similarly investigated; they were chosen from the same obstetrical service used by the subjects with rubella and were matched to them for maternal age, race, parity, and date of last menstrual period.

Initially, 769 women who contracted rubella were considered for the study, comprising about 10 percent of all rubella cases reported in females 15 to 44 years of age in New York City. However, 331 of those initially considered underwent therapeutic abortion and thereby eliminated themselves as candidates for surveillance; five women were either lost to follow-up before delivery or had multiple births, which disqualified them as participants. Fifty-two women experienced rubella during the later half of their pregnancies; these subjects were not included in the final data analysis. Of the remaining 381 cases of maternal rubella that occurred during the first half of gestation, 222 occurred in 1964 as a consequence of a major rubella epidemic that swept the United States during 1964 and 1965, and 159 occurred during the preceding seven years. The cases in both the epidemic and endemic periods were comparable with respect to maternal age, race, obstetrical history, and type of medical service. However, they differed somewhat in week of gestation at the onset of rubella. In analyzing the data, cases were further restricted to those in which rubella occurred within the first 20 weeks of gestation, because virtually no sequelae were noted in the children born to mothers who acquired rubella later than the twentieth week of pregnancy. The control group experienced

*M. Seigel, H.T. Fuerst, and V.F. Guince, "Rubella Epidemicity and Embryopathy: Results of a Long-Term Prospective Study." *Am. J. Dis. Child* 121:469–473, (1971).

virtually no sequelae that could be mistaken for congenitally acquired rubella. Table 10 summarizes findings from the 1964 epidemic.

It is obvious from this analysis of information acquired prospectively that the risk of congenital rubella is appreciable, particularly if the mother acquires the infection during the first trimester (first three months of pregnancy), for which the rate is 54.2 percent. The overall rate of 33.7 percent for the first 20 weeks of gestation is also substantial. In order to compare the epidemic year (1964) with the preceding nonepidemic years (1957–1963), it was necessary to adjust the rates to take into account the fact that the distribution by week of gestation at onset of rubella differed. The gestational-age-adjusted rate for the cases generated by the 1964 epidemic was 32 percent, compared to 22.5 percent for the preepidemic cases. The reason for this difference is not understood; perhaps the epidemic of 1964 was produced by a strain of rubella virus that was inherently more pathogenic than those prevalent before. In any case the data suffice for counseling a woman who contracts rubella in the first 20 weeks of her pregnancy concerning the probability of her having a congenitally damaged infant. Prospective investigations in other parts of the world, although differing in details of design, all yielded results comparable to those presented, thereby establishing the level of risk, which ranged from 50 to 60 percent in women exposed to rubella during the first trimester. Why 40 to 50 percent of such exposed women do not bear malformed babies is a question yet to be answered.

Even before the results of the several futuristically oriented investigations were known, virologists succeeded in growing rubella virus in tissue culture, and not long thereafter several live, attenuated rubella virus vaccine formulations were ready for testing under field conditions. One such study was conducted in Taiwan during the first major rubella epidemic that country had

Table 10
Major Congenital Malformations Following Maternal Rubella in 1964

Week of Gestation at Onset of Rubella	Number of Live Births	Major Congenital Defects			
		With Rubella Triad*	Without Rubella Triad**	Total No.	%
0–3	7	2	0	2	28.6
4–7	26	15	3	18	69.2
8–11	50	22	3	25	50.0
12–15	62	11	0	11	17.7
16–19	33	2	2	4	12.1
Total	178	52	8	60	33.7

*Congenital deafness, cardiac defects and cataracts, either singly or in combination with other malformations.
**Mental retardation or other major defects.

experienced in 10 years.* Because rubella had not been endemic in Taiwan preceding the epidemic, a large number of susceptible children had accumulated, making the situation ideal for vaccine testing.

After pilot studies that indicated that the vaccines to be evaluated were safe and largely free of undesirable side effects, four public primary schools, two in Taipei (population over one million) and two in Taichung (population just under 400,000), were selected for vaccine efficacy trials. Grades 1 through 4 were selected, because most fifth-grade children had been alive during the previous epidemic and about half of them had demonstrable rubella antibody. The combined enrollment of the first- to fourth-graders in the four schools was 15,000. Only males were included in the field trial so as not to deprive females of the known long-lasting immunity conferred by natural infection. The boys volunteered by their parents for inclusion in the trial were assigned to vaccine groups according to random permutations of five letters. Each of three rubella vaccine formulations was assigned one letter designation and the other two letters were assigned to poliovirus vaccine placebo. In order not to risk a disruption of the epidemic in the event the vaccine was effective in producing enough immunity soon enough to block person-to-person transmission (so called *herd immunity*), it was planned that not more than 30 percent of the boys in any classroom would receive rubella vaccine.

Subsequent to immunization, surveillance of clinical rubella was conducted in each school three times a week by a team of nurses trained to identify the rash. Table 11 reveals the results of this surveillance.

Table 11

Incidence of Rubella by School and Surveillance Group during the Fourth through Sixteenth Week after Immunization

	Taipei Schools		Taichung Schools	
Surveillance Group	Number of Children	Rubella Cases %	Number of Children	Rubella Cases %
Rubella vaccine 1	664	0.7	632	1.8
Rubella vaccine 2	660	1.9	427	1.4
Rubella vaccine 3	670	1.6	225	2.2
Poliovirus vaccine	1374	37.0	1367	19.0
Unvaccinated boys	1865	40.0	–	–
Unvaccinated girls	4732	45.0	2467	22.0
Total	9965		5118	

*R. Detels, J.T. Grayson, K.S.W. Kim, K.P. Chen, L. Gutman, J.K. Gale, and R.P. Beasley, "The Efficacy of HPV-77 Rubella Vaccine in Prevention of Disease." International Symposium of Rubella Vaccines. London 1968. *Symp. Series Immunobiol. Standard.*, Vol. II (New York, 1969) pp. 356–370.

It is clear from the table that the protection afforded by the three formulations of rubella vaccine was substantial when compared with the disease experience of the other groups.

A comparison of the protection afforded by each vaccine can be made conveniently by computing the protection rate (effectiveness, efficacy rate) for each, using the rate for the placebo group as a reference. For vaccines 1, 2, and 3, the protection rates were 95 percent, 94 percent, and 93 percent, respectively; each vaccine, therefore, may be deemed to be equally effective and of a high order. Other studies throughout the world yielded similar findings, thereby establishing rubella vaccine as a prophylactic modality for primary prevention of the disease.

Uses of Disease Rates

It should be apparent from the foregoing that disease rates provide knowledge of health-related phenomena that cannot be acquired by any other means. Disease rates depict disease occurrence in populations, and they are applicable to investigations of widely ranging purposes. These include assessing needs for medical facilities and programs, planning and evaluating programs for disease control and tests of new preventive and curative modalities, and studying disease etiology.

We have seen that the incidence rate of a disease in a group of people exposed to a factor is a measure of the *absolute risk* (or simply risk) of the disease in those exposed to that factor. The absolute risk is what a person exposed to a potentially harmful factor usually wants to know. This, of course, is only meaningful if it has been shown that this risk to the exposed is significantly greater than the risk to the unexposed. If this is the case, then a statistical association between the factor and the disease is said to exist. The *relative risk* is the measure of association commonly used to quantitate the strength of the association. It is of particular interest to those considering disease etiology.

Once a causal relationship between a disease and a factor has been established, then the absolute risk can be put in proper perspective for the person concerned about his exposure by considering the *excess risk* (sometimes called the attributable risk in the exposed). This is merely the rate in the exposed minus the rate in the nonexposed, and it is a measure of the amount of risk in the exposed that is due to the exposure.

If the proportion of a population that is exposed to a factor is known, then the *population attributable risk* (sometimes known simply as the attributable risk) can also be calculated. This is the proportion of the disease in the population that is due to the factor. This proportion (or percentage) is of value in determining the impact that a program to eliminate the factor would have on the overall disease problem in the population.

The absolute risk and the excess risk can be calculated only from studies in which disease incidence is measured. The relative risk and the population attributable risk can also be calculated from these kinds of investigations, and from case-control studies as well.

The relationship between cigarette smoking and lung cancer provides an example of these concepts. In one prospective study, the annual incidence rate of lung cancer per 1,000 population was found to be 1.30 for smokers (the absolute risk in smokers) and 0.07 for nonsmokers. The relative risk, therefore, is 18.6 (1.30/0.07), which means that the relationship between smoking and lung cancer is very strong (the risk in smokers is 18.6 times the risk in nonsmokers). The strength of this association, plus other considerations, strongly suggest that the association is a causal one (that is, that smoking is involved in the etiology of lung cancer).

The annual excess risk is 1.23 per 1,000 population (1.30-0.07). This means that smokers have this risk of lung cancer in excess of the risk to which they would be subjected if they did not smoke.

Finally, if 50 percent of a population is composed of people who smoke, then it can be calculated that 90 percent of the lung cancer in the population is due to smoking (if the above rates apply to this population). A program to eliminate smoking in the population would thus, in time, reduce by 90 percent the overall number of lung cancer cases.

These considerations of risk are summarized as follows:

Type of risk	Types of studies that can be used to measure risk type	Persons to which risk type is of interest
Absolute	prospective only	exposed person
Excess	prospective only	exposed person
Relative	prospective and case-control	person studying etiology
Population attributable	prospective and case-control	program planner

An understanding of these concepts by the practicing physician will aid him in intelligently advising his patients who are exposed to environmental hazards, in critically evaluating the medical literature that deals with considerations of etiology, and in planning programs of primary disease prevention.

Future use of disease rates for investigating new health-related phenomena can be expected from the fact that the population explosion, attended as it is by increasing urbanization, will engender a more complex physical environment, a more involved social milieu, and a more intense mental ambience, all of which will generate problems that will test the mettle of future epidemiologists.

Epidemiology and Statistics

Because epidemiology deals with rendering facts from figures, which are frequently presented in the form of tables or graphs, it may be construed by a casual observer as medical statistics, and to a degree, of course, it is. But it should be clear from the presentation up to this point that although epidemiologists use statistics, their primary interest and emphasis is focused on the distribution of health-related phenomena in human populations. By contrast, mathematically trained statisticans tend to concentrate on what can be done with numbers themselves; the biostatistician's forte is fitting mathematical models to biological phenomena in order to enhance the quantification process. As epidemiology has progressed into areas of inquiry of increasing complexity, the knowledge and skill of biostatisticians have become indispensable adjuncts to those of epidemiologists. This is reflected in an ever-increasing number of scientific papers coauthored by biostatisticians and epidemiologists; indeed, some biostatisticians, by virtue of their professional experience, consider themselves, with some justification, to be epidemiologists, and vice versa.

In this text, epidemiology has been presented as a discipline based on the use of disease rates, the computation and utilization of which require knowledge of ordinary arithmetic and only the most elementary algebra. These simple skills suffice for the bulk of epidemiological endeavor. On occasion, however, there is a need for use of descriptive statistics other than proportions. These include use of such parameters as means, standard deviations, medians, modes, and centiles, which are used to quantitate distributions.

At times a need arises for the application of statistical theory, so that the role of chance in producing a given result can be estimated. A variety of statistical tests are used to calculate precise probability values for random variation (chance). Such values, termed P values, range between 0 and 1 and express the likelihood with which observed results might have occurred on the basis of chance alone. The lower (closer to zero) the P value, the less likely it is that chance alone could account for observed differences in frequencies, means, proportions, and so forth. $P = 0.05$ may be interpreted as 1 chance in 20 that sampling error alone produced the results from which the P value was derived. Put another way, the odds are 19 to 1 against a result as extreme as that observed being due entirely to chance. $P < 0.05$ is a commonly used level of significance (5 percent), but its popularity hinges on nothing of substance; it is an arbitrary standard. One may just as well decide on a hedge against misinterpreting a chance result as a real one by adopting a level of significance of $P < 0.01$ or $P < 0.10$.

Statistical significance should not necessarily be equated with biological or medical significance. Observations can differ significantly or correlate highly but still be absurd from a biological or medical point of view. This is particularly likely to occur when multiple analyses and statistical tests of significance are made on subsets of the same data. As more and more such analyses are performed, the probability of encountering one exhibiting statistical significance purely by chance increases. Also, with samples of relatively large size, relatively small and biologically meaningless differences may test as statistically significant. Whether such an association has biological relevance must be decided from other evidence.

Also, lack of statistical significance of an association that makes biological sense may result from samples of inadequate size to yield statistical significance. Sample size is one of the terms that influences P values.

As epidemiologic investigations become increasingly comprehensive and complex, involving a large number of variables that interact in varying degree, biostatisticians find ample exercise for their talents in computer technology and the development of new and better methods of data anlysis and display.

The melding of the medical background of the epidemiologist with that of the mathematically oriented biostatistican has proved fruitful in the past and promises to continue to prosper in terms of providing knowledge of health-related phenomena in populations.

Disease Rates and Health

According to Terris, the major tasks of medicine, as originally conceived by Sigerist, embraced four separate components: the promotion of health, the prevention of illness, the restoration of the sick, and rehabilitation. Later, Leavell and Clark adopted and modified these components and called them levels of prevention, as follows:

Primary prevention
   Health promotion (dietary, hygiene, etc.)
   Specific protection (immunizations, vitamin and mineral supplements)

Secondary prevention
   Early recognition and treatment of disease

Tertiary prevention
   Disability limitation
   Rehabilitation

Of these five tasks, health promotion has received virtually no scientific attention comparable to that accorded the others, despite its obvious importance. Like epidemiology, health can be defined in many ways, none of which will satisfy everyone because the word health, from a semantic point of view, denotes an abstract condition that has no simple, single referent in the everyday world. Nevertheless, the World Health Organization has promulgated a definition that, from a philosophical point of view at least, is intended to express an ultimate goal that is worthy of pursuit. This definition maintains that health is a state of complete physical, social, and mental well-being, and not just the absence of disease. Health is portrayed in positive terms, as opposed to the absence of negative aspects. By definition, disease rates illuminate the health of populations negatively rather than positively. Because health is such an elusive object of investigation, little has been done on the epidemiology of health beyond speculation concerning the desirability of knowledge of factors that contribute, in a positive way, to physical, social, and mental well-being.

Health and disease may not be mutually exclusive states. Countless individuals who frequent doctors' offices and outpatient clinics for professional advice in the management of this or that chronic disease or disability lead otherwise happy and productive lives. The biographical literature is replete with examples of outstanding people whose physical, social, and mental well-being was of high caliber despite the stigma of disease or deformity. It seems reasonable to postulate, therefore, that health and disease can coexist in some individuals, but that health for most people implies the absence of at least recognizable forms of disease. The traditional dichotomization of health and disease is largely a matter of semantics.

If health is pictured simplistically as the coexistence of two fundamental attributes of well-being, namely, feeling and function, which are scaled in degree in both a positive and negative direction, then disease, with respect to the disease spectrum concept, must overlap into sectors that define various degrees of well-being. Figure 10 depicts the relationship just described on a pair of coordinates that demarcate four sectors of the correlation between feeling and function.

The figure indicates that the bulk of disease occupies the sector defined negatively with respect to both feeling and function—a condition experienced by virtually anyone who has been ill. But more importantly, the figure illustrates the overlapping of disease into the sectors where feeling or function, or both, are scaled positively, that is, approaching an optimal condition. The point to be emphasized here, as stated previously, is that health and disease are not necessarily mutually exclusive when health is defined in terms that reflect a sense of psychological well-being coincident with satisfactory performance in both social and physical aspects of living. Perhaps future generations of epidemiologists will be able to devise suitable rates for quantifying health so that positive steps can be taken in its promotion.

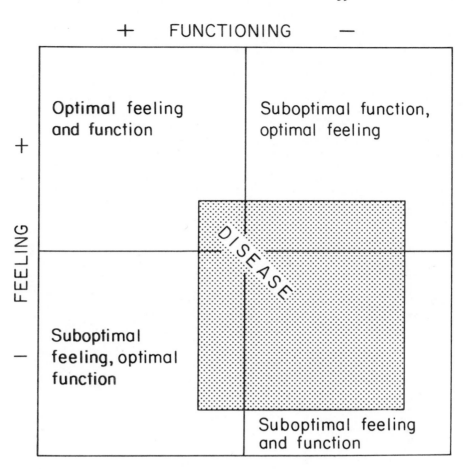

Figure 10. Feeling and Functioning as Definers of Health

Problems

Problem 1
The Disease Spectrum

Tables P-1 and P-2 show data from eight individuals who became ill approximately two days after exposure to the same child with stomach flu.

Table P-1. November 25: Hour of Symptom Onset, Estimated to Nearest Hour (24-hour clock)

Symptom and Signs	Patients							
	1	2	3	4	5	6	7	8
Malaise	9	9	9	10	12	16	8*	2*
Anorexia	9	9	9	10	12	22	8*	8*
Headache	–	?	–	9*	12	1*	8*	5*
Nausea	12	9	20	–	16	22	–	8*
Vomiting	14	10	20	–	–	23	–	–
Chills	–	?	23	–	16	23	–	17*
Abdominal pain	13	12	–	10	16	23	–	1*
Lassitude	18	9	12	10	12	16	8*	9*
Diarrhea	–	–	–	–	18	–	–	20
Myalgia	9	?	15	10	16	16	–	5*

*November 26 onset.

Table P-2. Duration of Each Symptom (in hours)

Symptom and Signs	Patients							
	1	2	3	4	5	6	7	8
Malaise	6	36	36	44	24	5	15	20
Anorexia	12	35	46	26	24	34	15	16
Headache	–	?	–	24	20	3	2	4
Nausea	3	36	7	–	9	12	–	11
Vomiting	1	30	7	–	–	1	–	–
Chills	–	?	8	–	9	4	–	2
Abdominal pain	5	24	–	22	7	20	–	3
Lassitude	3	36	34	44	24	38	15	12
Diarrhea	–	–	–	–	34	–	15	12
Myalgia	3	?	14	44	12	38	–	16

In view of the circumstances, it seems reasonable to assume that the eight individuals have the same disease. The tables reveal that a spectrum of clinical

61

responses and severity (inferable from duration of symptom) resulted. Most of the symptoms listed are subjective in character, and their presence must be ascertained from what a patient says. A few of the signs can be considered objective, some corroborating the presence of a symptom. The act of vomiting, which can be verified in various ways, supports the credibility of the complaint of nauseas.

Instructions and questions:

1. Inspect the data. Describe the spectrum of disease in terms of number, type, and duration of symptoms.
2. List the symptoms and signs in order of decreasing relative frequency.
3. Decide which symptom or sign or combination thereof might be the best indicator of a departure from a previous state of health, which could be used to index disease onset in time.
4. Calculate the mean duration of each symptom or sign and list them in rank order of duration, from longest to shortest.
5. Calculate the median duration of each symptom or sign and list them in rank order of duration, as above. The median is the point in time when 50 percent of the cases had occurred.
6. Which measure of central tendency, the mean or median, gives a better approximation of the number distributions in table P–2? Why?

Problem 2
Epidemic Curves

Incident cases of mumps occurring in an elementary school are listed in table P–3 by date of onset and grade. In the table, C = the case number, D = the date of onset, and G = the grade (K = kindergarten).

Table P–3.

C	D	G	C	D	G	C	D	G	C	D	G
1	Mar. 1	K	14	Apr. 2	6	27	Apr. 4	K	40	Apr. 6	4
2	16	K	15	2	1	28	5	1	41	6	1
3	16	K	16	2	1	29	5	1	42	6	3
4	17	K	17	2	1	30	5	2	43	6	3
5	18	1	18	3	3	31	5	2	44	6	2
6	18	K	19	3	K	32	5	2	45	6	2
7	18	K	20	4	K	33	5	4	46	7	4
8	18	K	21	4	1	34	5	2	47	7	5
9	18	K	22	4	4	35	5	2	48	7	2
10	19	1	23	4	1	36	5	3	49	7	2
11	22	K	24	4	3	37	5	1	50	8	4
12	31	K	25	4	K	38	5	1	51	8	5
13	Apr. 1	2	26	4	K	39	5	3	52	9	5

Construct a frequency histogram of incident cases by date of onset for each grade, and for the entire school as well, on graph paper, as illustrated in figure P-1. Use the lowest line for the composite epidemic curve, that is, for the entire school.

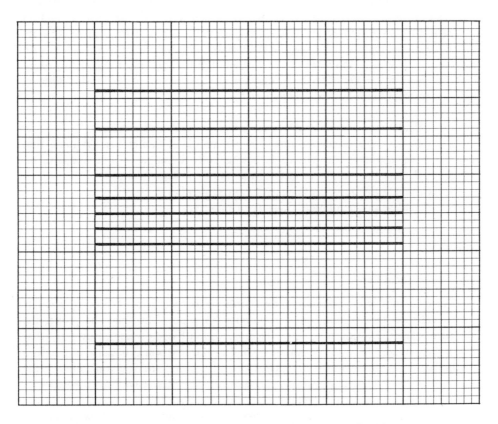

Figure P-1. Graph Layout for Frequency Histogram in Problem 2.

Questions:

1. From the appearance of the epidemic curves, describe how the disease apparently spread through the school. What are the most probable reasons for the observed pattern?
2. From the composite epidemic curve, estimate the incubation period of mumps.
3. How does this curve differ from that of an epidemic due to exposure to a common nonhuman source of infection, such as a polluted water supply or contaminated food?

Problem 3
Incidence and Prevalence Rates

Figure P-2 summarizes a disease outbreak. The time of disease onset, length of illness, and outcome (recovery or death) of each case is shown. This outbreak occurred in a remote community of 502 persons (all male, between 20 and 55 years of age) employed by a logging contractor. None of the employees were native to the region, and it may be assumed that this was their first encounter with the disease agent. As shown in the diagram, the first case occurred on August 22 and the last on October 2. Altogether, 23 persons experienced the disease.
Perform the following calculations:

1. Calculate the overall attack rate.
2. Calculate the incidence rate for the month of September. (Assume that after recovery, the patient is permanently immune to a second attack.)
3. Calculate the prevalence rate for the month of September.
4. Calculate the point prevalence rate on September 7.
5. Calculate the case fatality ratio (percentage).

Problem 4
Conventional Rates

For epidemiological purposes, rates should be as specific as technically possible to enhance their utilization as a population probe; the finer the probe, the greater the resolution of a particular observation based on rates. However, what is theoretically ideal often cannot be had in the real world because of practical limitations in the manner in which data are recorded and the availability of the needed raw material. Accordingly, a number of indices have been devised over the years, largely on the premise that they represent the best available measurement tools. Many of these indices have become known as *conventional rates*. Some are not true rates, however, in that individuals in the numerator are not contained in the denominator.

Examine the following list of conventional rates and write a short commentary on the relationship of the numerator to the denominator for each, and its possible uses and limitations.

1. Crude death rate $= \dfrac{\text{No. of deaths in a year}}{\text{Mid-year population}} \times 1000$

2. Crude birth rate $= \dfrac{\text{No. of live births in a year}}{\text{Mid-year population}} \times 1000$

65

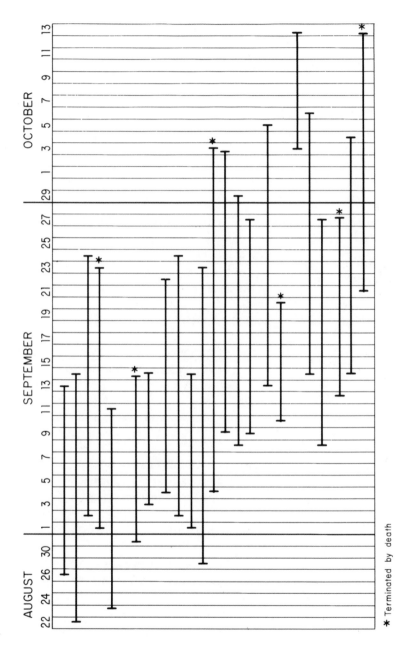

* Terminated by death

Figure P-2. Diagram for Problem 3.

3. Infant mortality rate $= \dfrac{\text{No. of infant deaths in a year}}{\text{No. of live births in the same year}} \times 1000$

(infants are defined as children less than 365 days old)

4. Neonatal mortality rate $= \dfrac{\text{No. of neonatal deaths in a year}}{\text{No. of live births in the same year}} \times 1000$

(The neonatal period is the first 28 days of life)

5. Postneonatal mortality rate $= \dfrac{\text{No. of postneonatal deaths in a year}}{\text{No. of live births in the same year}} \times 1000$

(The postneonatal period includes the 29th through the 365th day of life)

6. Stillbirth rate (fetal death rate) $= \dfrac{\text{No. of still births in a year}}{\text{No. of live births and stillbirths in the same year}} \times 1000$

(A stillbirth is a baby born dead after 28 or more weeks of gestation)

7. Perinatal mortality rate $= \dfrac{\text{No. of perinatal deaths in a year}}{\text{No. of live births and stillbirths in the same year}} \times 1000$

(The perinatal period is from the 28th week of gestation through the first week of life)

8. Maternal mortality rate $= \dfrac{\text{No. of deaths due to deliveries and complications of pregnancy, childbirth, and the puerperium in a year}}{\text{No. of live births in the same year}} \times 1000$

9. Annual cause-of-death rate $= \dfrac{\text{No. of deaths from a specified cause that occurred among the population of a given geographic area during a given year}}{\text{Mid-year total population of the given geographic area during the same year}} \times 100{,}000$

10. Annual cause-specific Morbidity rate $= \dfrac{\text{No. of cases of a specified disease that occurred among the population of a given geographic area during a given year}}{\text{Mid-year total population of the given geographic area during the same year}} \times 100{,}000$

Problem 5
A Descriptive Study

The age distribution pattern shown in table P–4 was associated with an epidemic of measles in a population living on a remote island. These are real data collected in 1846.

Table P–4.

Age (years)	Number of Persons	Number with Measles	Incidence Rate (%)
1	198	154	77.8
1–9	1440	1117	77.7
10–19	1525	1183	77.6
20–29	1470	1140	77.6
30–39	842	653	77.6
40–59	1519	1178	77.6
60–79	752	583	77.5
80+	118	92	78.0

Answer the following questions:

1. What is the usual distribution of measles incidence by age?
2. What inference can you draw concerning susceptibility to measles from the data shown in the table?
3. What inference can you draw concerning prior exposure to measles from the data shown in the table?
4. How can one account for the fact that approximately one-quarter of the population in every age group appears to have escaped infection?

Problem 6
Sensitivity and Specificity

Although the concepts of sensitivity and specificity are usually applied to diagnostic laboratory tests, they are equally valid for other sorts of tests that indicate the presence or absence of disease. These may be tests designed to elicit certain physical signs of disease by examination (specific heart murmurs, neuro-logical defects, tendency to hemorrhage or questions aimed at uncovering symptoms or symptom complexes.

Suppose that a short psychometric questionnaire, devised to detect undiag-nosed cases of personality disorders, was found after several trials in different clinics to have a sensitivity of 25 percent and a specificity of 99 percent.

Questions:

1. Would this questionnaire be more useful as a clinical or public health tool? Explain.
2. If 262 persons, half of whom did not, in fact, have a personality disorder, were tested, how many false negatives would result? How many false positives?
3. What are the adverse consequences of using a test of low sensitivity to screen for a disease?
4. What are the adverse consequences of using a test of low specificity to screen for a disease?

Problem 7
Rate Adjustment

Figure 8 in the text indicates that the age-specific death rates for Malays in West Malaysia exceed those for residents of Washington State for every age group by a substantial margin. Yet the overall or crude death rate for Washingtonians exceeds that for Malays (8.8 per thousand versus 7.6 per thousand). The reason is that, as shown in Figure 1, the two populations differ remarkably in age com-position. Washington State has proportionately more older people whose rates of dying are high compared to people at younger ages.

Perform calculations and answer the following questions:

1. From the data in table P-5, calculate the age-standardized (adjusted) death rate for Malays, using the population of Washington State as the standard population.

Table P-5. Age Standardization Computation

Age Groups (years)	Mortality Rates* (Malays)	Washington State Population	Expected Deaths
0–4	15.0	280,472	_____
5–14	1.6	677,339	_____
15–24	1.6	625,867	_____
25–34	2.7	432,102	_____
35–44	4.3	373,848	_____
45–54	9.9	392,654	_____
55–64	24.9	304,906	_____
65+	70.1	322,061	_____
Total		3,409,169	_____

*Deaths per 1000 population.

This age-adjusted death rate may now be compared with the overall rate for Washington State. The latter rate does not have to be age-adjusted for this comparison because the population of Washington State was (arbitrarily) chosen as the standard population for the age adjustment of the Malay rate.

2. In contrast to the crude Malay rate, how does the age-adjusted Malay rate compare with the crude Washington State rate?

3. The total rate for Malays of 7.6 per 1,000 does not equal the average of the age-specific rates shown in table P-5, which is 16.3 per 1,000. Explain.

4. Disease rates can be adjusted for more than one factor. When comparing rates in two populations, they should be adjusted for any factor that both influences the rate under consideration and is distributed differently in the two populations. For example, it can be seen from Figure 9 in the text that sex as well as age influences mortality rates in both Malays and Washingtonians. If the two populations differ in their sex composition, this will influence a comparison of the overall rates for the two populations. Table P-6 contains the data required to standardize for age and sex simultaneously. Calculate the overall mortality rate for Malays standardized against the Washington State population for both age and sex. What conclusion can be drawn from the result?

Table P–6

Age Groups (years)	Mortality per 1,000 Malay Males	Washington State Male Population	Expected Male Deaths
0–4	16.5	142,996	_____
5–14	1.6	346,363	_____
15–24	1.6	317,474	_____
25–34	2.4	218,091	_____
35–44	4.3	185,792	_____
45–54	10.5	193,989	_____
55–64	25.9	150,099	_____
65+	72.5	139,023	_____
Total	8.0	1,693,827	_____

Age Groups (years)	Mortality per 1,000 Malay Females	Washington State Female Population	Expected Female Deaths
0–4	13.4	137,476	_____
5–14	1.5	330,976	_____
15–24	1.7	308,393	_____
25–34	2.9	214,011	_____
35–44	4.3	188,056	_____
45–54	9.3	198,665	_____
55–64	23.8	154,807	_____
65+	67.5	183,038	_____
Total	5.1	1,715,422	_____

Problem 8
A Prospective Study

An epidemiologic study of the common cold was conducted in a series of American households. Among other things, the numbers of secondary cases that occurred subsequent to a primary case in each household under study was ascertained during one winter. Data from 664 households are shown in table P–7. The residents of these households have been categorized according to the degree of crowding in their household. Assume that there was one primary case in each household.

Table P-7.

Degree of Crowding in Households	Number of Households	Number of Residents	Total Number of Cases
Most	241	964	399
Intermediate	242	968	373
Least	181	724	307

Instructions and questions:

1. Calculate the secondary attack rate for residents of the three groups of households.
2. Do the results of this study suggest that the spread of colds in households is influenced by degree of crowding? Give two reasons for your answers.

Problem 9
A Case-Control Study

A number of studies have provided evidence that herpes simplex virus type-2 (HSV-2) may be a cause of cancer of the cervix. One study involved measuring humoral HSV-2 antibodies in a series of 52 cervical cancer patients and in a comparable series of 52 women without this disease. Forty-three of the cases and 18 of the controls were found to have measurable HSV-2 antibodies.

Questions:

1. Calculate the relative risk of cervical cancer in women with HSV-2 antibodies (relative to women without these antibodies).
2. Do the study results show an association between cervical cancer and HSV-2 antibodies?
3. Are these results sufficient to establish that HSV-2 is a cause of cervical cancer? If not, what are some alternative interpretations of these findings.

Problem 10
An Experimental Study

In his book *Vitamin C and the Common Cold*, Nobel prize-winner (for chemistry and peace) Linus Pauling advanced the thesis that ascorbic acid in large daily doses (1 to 3 grams daily) could prevent upper respiratory infections. Claims made in the book were highly speculative and generated considerable skepticism

in scientific circles. Subsequently, several carefully designed double-blind prophylactic trials were conducted to evaluate properly Pauling's enthusiastic
endorsement, which was based on rather flimsy scientific evidence. One such
study* was carefully designed and conducted with a view to making the investigation as objective as possible. The following two tables summarize the results
of the study: table P-8 deals with disease episodes and table P-9 with days of
illness—two ways of assessing potential benefit during a 14-week period.

Table P-8. Attack Rates by Study Group

Group	Number of Respiratory Illnesses	Number of Children	Attack Rate (%)
Vitamin C	35	321	10.9
Placebo	40	320	12.5

Table P-9. Sick-Day Rates by Study Group

Group	Number of Sick Days	Number of Days of Observation	Days Sick (%)
Vitamin C	325	2007	16.2
Placebo	415	1922	21.6

Questions:

1. From table P-8, calculate the protection rate against illness.
2. From table P-9, calculate the protection rate against sick days.
3. Comment on the efficacy of vitamin C prophylaxis of respiratory illness on
   the basis of this evidence.

Problem 11
Classification of Investigations

Classify each of the following five studies by marking the appropriate cell in
the blank table at the end of the series.

  1. A series of consecutive admissions to the hospital of patients with a
specific disease, the occurrence of which is suspected of being influenced by

---

*J.L. Coulehan, K.S. Reisinger, K.D. Rogers, and D.W. Bradley, "Vitamin C. Prophylaxis
in a Boarding School," *New Eng. J. Med.* 290:6–10 (1974).

personal contact, is used to identify relatives and friends with whom they have consorted during the preceding four years and who live in the area served by the hospital. Records of the hospital are then searched for the names of these relatives and friends who might have been admitted during the four-year period with the same condition. The incidence rate of the disease in the relatives and friends is compared with that for the entire community for evidence that the incidence is higher in close associates than in the community at large.

2.   The parents of children in several classrooms of an elementary school are requested to relate whether their child has ever had mumps. A random sample of those with a negative history were tested serologically for mumps antibody; all were negative. The children with a negative mumps history were than randomly allocated to one of two groups. The first group received live attenuated mumps virus vaccine, and the other group received a suitably disguised placebo. An outbreak of mumps occurred in the school a few months later. After it had subsided, mumps attack rates were computed for the two groups.

3.   Residents of three villages with three different types of water supply were asked to participate in a survey to identify cholera carriers. Because several cholera deaths had occurred in the recent past, virtually everyone present at the time submitted to examination. The proportion of residents in each village who were carriers was computed and compared.

4.   Some babies born to mothers with proved leprosy were found being reared by their natural mother, and some were found being reared in foster homes. Over the following ten years, careful measurements were made periodically in both groups of babies for evidence of disease.

5.   From hospital charts of 40 patients diagnosed as having dengue fever, it was noted that a large proportion had fasted during the two-week period preceding onset. To determine if fasting is associated with clinical dengue, a series of 40 patients with nondengue febrile illness was collected, matched for age, sex, and race to the dengue patients. The hospital charts of these patients were then reviewed also to determine fasting prior to their illness.

				Study Number		
Avenue of Investigation		1	2	3	4	5
Prevalence						
Historically Oriented	Nonconcurrent prospective					
	case-control					
Futuristic cohort	Concurrent prospective					
	Experimental					

Answers to Problems

Problem 1
The Disease Spectrum

1. The clinical response varied. Patients reported as few as four symptoms that were generally mild (and subjective), and as many as nine symptoms and signs that included indices of severe discomfort. For example, patient 7 had only vague feelings of discomfort and weakness, with some headache and loss of appetite, which lasted a relatively short period of time, while patient 2 had abdominal pains and vomiting that lasted over two days.

2. Malaise 8/8; anorexia 8/8; lassitude 8/8; nausea 6/8; abdominal pain 6/8; myalgia 6/8; headache 5/8; vomiting 4/8; chills 4/8; diarrhea 2/8.

3. Everyone experienced malaise (not feeling well in a nonspecific way), anorexia (loss of appetite), and lassitude (weakness), and therefore any one of these symptoms could be used arbitrarily. However, malaise and anorexia correspond most closely with respect to time of onset (probably because many patients equated the two symptoms), and tended to occur earlier than lassitude. Therefore, either of these symptoms, or whichever occurred first, would best serve as the indicator of the time of onset of disease.

4. Anorexia 209/8 = 26.1; lassitude 206/8 = 25.8; malaise 186/8 = 23.2; Diarrhea 46/2 = 23.0; myalgia 127/6 = 21.2; abdominal pain 81/6 = 13.5; nausea 78/6 = 13.0; headache 53/5 = 10.6; vomiting 39/4 = 9.8; chills 23/4 = 5.8.

5. Lassitude 29; anorexia 25; diarrhea 23; malaise 22; myalgia 15; abdominal pain 13.5; nausea 10; chills 6; vomiting 4; headache 4.

6. The two measures yield results that are comparable for the most part, although the ranking is shifted somewhat. The mean values for nausea and vomiting are higher than the median because of the single high figure in each distribution, which influences the mean but not the median. The median is the better statistic to use when the distribution is highly skewed (not symmetrical).

Problem 2
Epidemic Curves

1. The disease was introduced into the school by a child in kindergarten, who served as the source of infection for seven other cases in kindergarten and two in the first grade. These individuals, in turn, were the source of infection for the remainder of the cases. Also, at each successive year of age, as represented by grade in school, there are fewer cases, that is, K(15), 1(12), 2(10), 3(6), 4(5), 5(3), 6(1). See figure A-1.

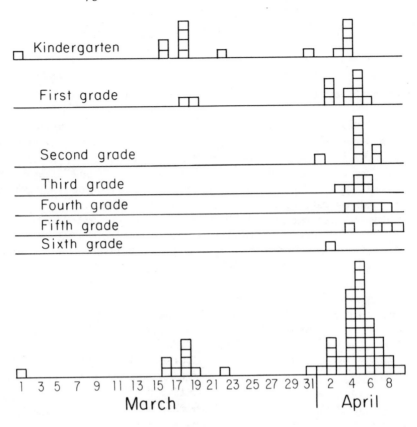

Figure A-1. Distribution of Mumps Cases by Date of Output (Problem 2).

The younger the child, the more likely it is that she or he has not yet encountered mumps virus, because of a restricted social environment. At least one sixth-grade pupil in this school was still susceptible, but most of his peers were probably immune. Exposure of all grades is facilitated by contact in hallways and contact during play periods, lunch periods, and on school buses. Not all such contacts are effective with respect to viral transmission, however.

2. From the index case on March 1, the shortest period was 16 days and the longest 22 days; the most common was 18 days (the mode or peak of the first wave). The peak of the subsequent generation of cases was 19 days after the mode of the first wave.

3. This is a *propagated epidemic*, in which the disease is transmitted from person to person by close contact of diseased and susceptible individuals. In a common-source epidemic, two patterns may result. If the exposure is at a single point in time (as is often the situation in food poisoning),

then a unimodal epidemic curve will be observed, usually without the occurrence of subsequent waves of cases after the initial wave. If the exposure is over a prolonged period of time (as in many instances of drinking-water contamination), then cases will also occur over a prolonged period of time, but will not occur in discrete waves (generations of cases), as in this mumps epidemic.

Problem 3
Incidence and Prevalence Rates

1. Overall attack rate = 23/502 = 4.6 percent.
2. September incidence rate = 17/497 = 3.4 percent. Note that the five cases with onset in August are subtracted from the denominator because these five people were not at risk in September by virtue of already having had the disease.
3. Period prevalence rate for September = 22/502 = 4.4 percent. All but one were ill at some time during the month of September. For prevalence rates, the denominator need not be corrected, because risk of acquiring disease is not at issue.
4. Point prevalence rate on September 7 = 12/502 = 2.4 percent.
5. Case fatality ratio = 6/23 × 100 = 26 percent.

Problem 4
Conventional Rates

1. *Crude death rate.* This rate meets the epidemiological criteria of a rate, provided that it is understood that the deceased persons comprising the numerator were living members of the population during the year in question. Vital statisticians will often tabulate deaths two ways: by residence and by occurrence. Deaths by residence usually include individuals who happened to die while away from their area of residence as well as those who die while in residence. Deaths by occurrence include all such events in a population without regard to location of official residence.
2. *Crude birth rate.* In one sense this rate falls short of being epidemiologically acceptable because the production of babies is contingent primarily upon the number of females in a population; males are accessories to the phenomenon. Furthermore, pregnancy is biologically restricted to an age range conventionally reckoned as 15 to 49 years or 15 to 44 years. A measure called the *general fertility rate* is defined as the number of live births in a year divided by the number of women of reproductive age in the mid-year population times 1,000.

3. *Infant mortality rate.* This is a true rate. However, the bulk of infant mortality occurs within the first week of life (approximately three-fourths of all infant deaths). Because most of the babies comprising the numerator of this rate are at one end of the infancy age range, this rate is a relatively gross instrument for indicating the risk of dying throughout the period of infancy.

4. *Neonatal mortality rate.* This is a true rate. By restricting the numerator events to a narrower age range, this rate provides greater fidelity for perceiving the force of infant mortality than does the infant mortality rate.

5. *Postneonatal mortality rate.* This rate is simply the complement of the neonatal mortality rate; together they comprise the infant mortality rate.

6. *Stillbirth rate.* This is a true rate. The proper denominator for fetal deaths is the number of pregnancies that continued to the 28th week of gestation or beyond, which is achieved by adding the stillbirths to the live births for the denominator.

7. *Perinatal mortality rate.* Epidemiologically, this rate makes sense. It was originally contrived to quantify the lethality that occurs during late pregnancy, childbirth, and very early infancy, so that obstetricians and pediatricians would have an index of the effect of their efforts at medical management during this critical period.

8. *Maternal mortality rate.* Althouth technically this is not a rate, the number of live births used as a denominator will approximate the number of women at risk to the conditions specified in the numerator. Because stillbirths are not included, the denominator will be shy a few individuals who might be included in the numerator. This underestimation is offset by the fact that multiple births (twins, triplets) will tend to inflate the denominator.

9. *Annual cause-of-death rate.* This is a true rate. However, those causes of death peculiar to certain demographic segments of society are represented only very grossly by this rate. If a cause of death primarily affects older people, one sex, or certain workers, for example, the inclusion of the entire population in the denominator dilutes the proportion such that the annual cause-of-death rate provides an uncertain measure for purposes of comparison unless the populations being compared are similar with respect to the relevant segments.

10. *Annual cause-specific morbidity rate.* Comments similar to those in number 9 above, are pertinent here. Childhood diseases expressed in terms of the whole population obviously become misrepresented by using the whole population as a denominator; school enrollment figures would provide a closer approximation. Venereal diseases would be more properly put in perspective if only persons in the age range in which substantial sexual promiscuity occurs constituted the denominator.

Problem 5
A Descriptive Study

1. The incidence is low in infancy and increases progressively during the pre-school and primary school years such that, by the age of 15 years, approximately 80 percent of the population is immune.
2. Susceptibility differed radically from the usual in that susceptibility appears to have been high at all ages.
3. There probably had been no encounter with measles virus by this population for more than 80 years.
4. Several possibilities exist:
   a. A constant proportion of people in each age group had inapparent infections. This is unlikely. Infections that are inapparent tend to vary with age, and it is now known that measles virus results in a lower proportion of inapparent infections than suggested by these data.
   b. Not everyone on the island may have been exposed. Family enclaves may have been isolated from the epidemic.
   c. Some of the population may have been immune by virtue of having been previously infected while off the island. This is not likely, however, because children were not more susceptible than adults at the time of the epidemic, and yet adults would be the ones most likely to have traveled in the past and contracted measles.
   d. Not all cases may have been counted. This is a possibility, but it is unlikely that the same proportion of cases in every age group would have been underascertained.
   e. Epidemic spread of measles subsides when a substantial proportion of susceptibles have converted to immune by virtue of having had the disease. As immunes accumulate, they serve as blocks to transmissions to the susceptibles remaining in the population. Several studies demonstrate that when a population becomes largely immune, measles spread tends to cease. This phenomenon is known as *herd immunity* and is a plausible explanation for incidence rates of less than 100 percent.

Problem 6
Sensitivity and Specificity

1. A testing instrument with a sensitivity of but 25% would miss 75% of the cases of personality disorder in a population; this high proportion of false negatives would discourage a public health application. However, in a clinical setting in which the primary focus is on diagnosis of individual

patients, a positive test would virtually confirm the presence of the disorder because only 1% of those without the disorder would be expected to have a positive result. On the other hand, a negative test would not exclude (rule out) the disorder.

2. In the following table, the 33 true positives resulted from the calculation $0.25 \times 131 = 32.75$. This rounds to 33. By subtracting 33 from 131, one obtains 98 false negatives (diseased people who were missed). Similarly, $0.99 \times 131 = 129.69$, rounded to 130 true negatives, and but 1 false positive (well person called diseased).

Personality Disorder	Questionnaire Result		
	Positive	Negative	Totals
Yes	33	98	131
No	1	130	131
Totals	34	228	262

3. A test of low sensitivity will fail to detect many of the cases, thus giving those missed a false sense of security. If early detection can lead to early treatment that can alter the course of disease (such as with certain cancers), then the lives of missed cases may be put in jeopardy by using an insensitive screening test.

4. A test of low specificity will erroneously label well individuals as ill. The consequences of such false alarm can be serious. The medical care system may be overloaded by people seeking additional diagnostic and treatment services, and well individuals may be subjected to the unnecessary expense, discomfort, and even danger of additional diagnostic tests or unwarranted treatments. Iatrogenic disease may result where previously there was no disease.

Problem 7
Rate Adjustment

1. Computation of age standardization:

Age Groups (years)	Expected Deaths
0–4	4,207
5–14	1,084
15–24	1,001
25–34	1,167
35–44	1,608
45–54	3,887
55–64	7,592
65+	22,576
Total	43,122

Overall death rate for Malays standardized for age against the population of Washington State $= \dfrac{43,122}{3,409,169} \times 1,000 = 12.6/1,000$

2. Standardization for age has reversed the relative order of magnitude of the overall death rates. *Crude death rate comparison*: Malays 7.6/1,000; Washingtonians 8.8/1,000. *After adjustment for age*: Malays 12.6/1,000; Washingtonians 8.8/1,000.

3. The total death rate results from the sum of all deaths, regardless of age, divided by the total number comprising the population. Each age-specific rate, if considered in original fractional form, has a different denominator. Fractions cannot be added unless numerator adjustments are made in the process of conversion to a common denominator. Because the age-specific rates were not converted to a common denominator in their original fraction form, their sum will violate the "fraction addition rule".

4. Computation of Adjustment for Age and Sex:

Age Groups (years)	Expected Male Deaths	Expected Female Deaths
0–4	2,359	1,842
5–14	554	496
15–24	508	524
25–34	523	621
35–44	799	809
45–54	2,037	1,848
55–64	3,888	3,684
65+	10,079	12,355
Total	20,747	22,179

Overall mortality rate for Malays standardized against the population of Washington State for both age and sex

$$= \dfrac{20,747 + 22,179}{1,693,827 + 1,715,422} \times 1,000$$

$$= \dfrac{42,926}{3,409,249} \times 1,000$$

$$= 12.6/1,000$$

Standardizing for both age and sex yields an adjusted rate that is virtually the same as the rate adjusted for age alone. The reason for this is that the two populations did not differ markedly in sex composition.

Problem 8
A Prospective Study

1. Calculation of secondary attack rates is demonstrated in the following table.

	(1)	(2)	(3)
Degree of Crowding in Households	Number of Households	Number of Residents	Number of Residents at Risk
Most	241	964	723
Intermediate	242	968	726
Least	181	724	543

	(4)	(5)	(6)
Degree of Crowding in Households	Number of Cases	Number of Secondary Cases	Secondary Attack Rate (%)
Most	399	158	21.9
Intermediate	373	131	18.0
Least	307	126	23.2

    a.   The number of residents at risk of exposure to a primary case is the total number of residents minus the number of primary cases. Because there is one primary case per household, the number at risk in column (3) equals the number in column (2) minus the number in column (1).

    b.   The number of secondary cases is the total number of cases minus the number of primary cases, which is derived by subtracting the numbers in column (1) from the numbers in column (4).

    c.   The secondary attack rate, then, is the numbers in column (5) divided by the numbers in column (3), expressed as a percent.

2. No, these results do not suggest that crowding influences the spread of colds in households. There are two reasons for this:

    a.   The differences between the three secondary attack rates are small (and could have occurred by chance alone).

    b.   There is no progressive increase in attack rates with degree of crowding.

Problem 9
A Case-Control Study

1. The relative risk (RR) is calculated from data in the following table.

HSV-2

HSV-2 Antibodies	Cases	Controls
Present	43	18
Absent	9	34
Total	52	52

$$RR = \frac{43 \times 34}{9 \times 18} = 9.02$$

2. These results indicate a strong statistical association between HSV-2 antibodies and cervical cancer.

3. These results alone are not sufficient proof that HSV-2 in a cause of cervical cancer. Alternative interpretations include:

a. Women with cervical cancer are more susceptible to HSV-2 infections. In this example, the case-control approach does not provide information as to whether the infection preceded or followed the cancer.

b. An unknown factor is the cause of cervical cancer, and HSV-2 virus is associated with the occurrence of this factor. This could result in the observation of a spurious association between HSV-2 antibodies and cervical cancer.

Problem 10
An Experimental Study

The protection rate is calculated from the formula:

$$(1 - \text{rate for vitamin C/rate for placebo}) \times 100$$

1. $(1 - 10.9/12.5) \times 100 = (1 - 0.87) \times 100 = 13$ percent.
2. $(1 - 16.2/21.6) \times 100 = (1 - 0.75) \times 100 = 25$ percent.
3. From this evidence it appears that vitamin C may afford some protection against acquiring an acute respiratory tract illness. It appears to be more effective in reducing the number of sick days, suggesting that severity of illness may be reduced. However, neither set of rates is statistically significant. The study is therefore inconclusive, that is, chance alone could have produced the results found.

Problem 11
Classification of Investigations

Avenue of Investigation		Study Number				
		1	2	3	4	5
Prevalence				X		
Historically oriented	Nonconcurrent prospective	X				
	Case-control					X
Futuristic cohort	Concurrent prospective				X	
	Experimental		X			

Specimen Examination
Questions

The following table indicates results of testing native Alaskans for antibody to *Toxoplasma gondii*.

Age of Time of Testing (years)	Women		Men	
	Number Tested	Number Positive	Number Tested	Number Positive
15–24	171	27	59	10
25–34	44	9	32	5
35–64	35	12	25	8
All ages	250	48	116	23

1. This study should be classified as (choose one):
   A. An incidence study
   B. An historical cohort study
   C. A case-control study
   D. A cross-sectional study
2. For comparison with overall rates for other populations these data should be (choose one):
   A. Adjusted for age
   B. Adjusted for sex
   C. Adjusted for both age and sex
   D. Not adjusted
3. One can infer from these data that (choose one):
   A. The incidence of toxoplasmosis infection increases with advancing years
   B. Males have the same risk as females of acquiring infections by *T. gondii*.
   C. Antibody prevalence is distributed approximately equally between the sexes
   D. None of the above
4. Inference: The risk of infection by *T. gondii* among natives residing in the arctic and subarctic regions of Alaska increases progressively with age.
   A. The inference is correct
   B. The inference is incorrect because the inference concerning risk is based on the incidence data
   C. The inference is incorrect because cohort effect could account for the results
   D. The inference is incorrect because of strong participant bias

Clinically inapparent hypothyroidism occurs in newborn babies at a rate of 1 per 6,000 live births. The condition can only be detected early by measuring the concentration of thyroxine or thyroid-stimulating hormone in the blood. Concentrations below some arbitrarily set figure are interpreted as a positive test result, while those above that figure are considered negative.

Each test costs $5.00. Half of the babies with the disease have a negative test. The proportion of babies who are classified by the test results as negative at birth but later develop signs and symptoms of the disease is not known. Appropriate treatment of infants who indeed have this disorder at birth will prevent both physical and mental retardation. Many pediatricians advocate publicly financed screening programs so that newborns with the defect can be identified and treated.

5. The rate cited (1 per 6,000 live births) is an example of (choose one):
   A. A crude incidence rate
   B. An age-specific incidence
   C. A period prevalence rate
   D. A variant of a point prevalence rate
6. How many newly born babies would have to be tested to identify correctly ten infants with clinically inapparant hypothyroidism at birth?
   A. 20   B. 3,000   C. 120,000   D. 60,000
7. What is the test specificity in this instance?
   A. 100%   B. 50%   C. 0%   D. Unknown
8. Treatment of newly born babies with hypothyroidism would fall into which one of the following classifications?
   A. Primary prevention
   B. Secondary prevention
   C. Tertiary prevention
   D. None of the above
9. At $5.00 per test and a low case-finding yield, the cost-to-benefit ratio of a public screening program would obviously be enormous. Which one of the following would be the least appropriate response to this problem?
   A. Set up a statewide screening program immediately
   B. Improve the test sensitivity and determine its specificity
   C. Expect that most instances of hypothyroidism in the newborn will be clinically recognizable on subsequent routine examinations during infancy and will be treated effectively
   D. Seek to develop other tests that can be used in conjunction with the tests currently available so that case classification will be more precise, although more expensive
10. From the relationships shown in figure E-1, select the correct interpretation from the following: I. If the disease duration is constant, the prevalence rate would decrease; II. If the disease duration is constant, the prevalence rate would also remain constant; III. The case fatality ratio is decreasing; IV. The case fatality ratio is increasing.

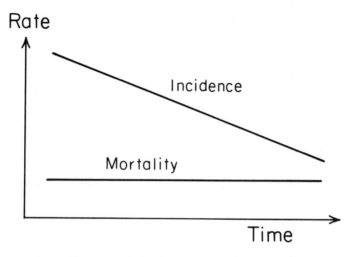

Figure E-1. Graph for Examination Question 10.

A. I and III are correct
B. I and IV are correct
C. II and III are correct
D. II and IV are correct

11. In a field trial of swine flu vaccine, either the vaccine or an identical-appearing placebo was administered to a group of 1,000 healthy volunteers, using double-blind procedures and random assignment of persons to treatment groups. All volunteers were followed during the subsequent six months by means of weekly telephone calls to determine their health status. During this time, a considerable number of cases of swine flu were documented in members of the general population by the laboratory of the health department that served the community in which the trial was conducted. For the purpose of the trial, flu was defined as any episode of acute febrile respiratory illness (AFRI). The following data were collected during the trial:

Treatment Group	Number of Persons	Number of Episodes of AFRI
Vaccine	492	53
Placebo	508	102

Based on these data, what was the protection rate for those vaccinated?
A. 6%   B. 12%   C. 46%   D. 73%

12. A new test to measure serum cholesterol concentration was evaluated as follows: A single blood specimen was drawn from each of 50 medical students. The serum was then separated from the blood cells and divided

into two aliquots (portions). Each aliquot was given a different code number, and the new test was then used to determine the cholesterol level in all 100 aliquots by a technician who was unaware of which aliquots came from which student. The levels of cholesterol in the two aliquots from each of the 50 specimens were then compared. This procedure provided the data that could be used to measure the tests: I. sensitivity; II. validity; III. specificity; IV. reliability; V. predictive value.

    A. I and III are correct

    B. II and IV are correct

    C. V is correct

    D. IV is correct

13. The test in question 12 was also used to make a single measurement of the cholesterol in 10 artificial samples that contained different known amounts of cholesterol. This procedure provided the data that could be used to measure the following:

    A. Validity

    B. Reliability

    C. Predictive value

    D. False positive rate

14. A case-control study of breast cancer was conducted to determine if there was a relationship of this disease to use of the antihypertensive drug reserpine. A total of 33 cases and 97 controls were studied; 15 of the cases and 30 of the controls were found to have used reserpine previously. Based on these data, the relative risk of breast cancer associated with prior reserpine use is:

    A. 0.50   B. 1.47   C. 1.86   D. 3.15

15. In 1970, 20 percent of 200 laboratory-confirmed cases of Salmonellosis in King County originated in families having a pet turtle. This is an example of (choose one):

    A. A case series study

    B. An incidence study

    C. A prevalence study

    D. A cohort study

16. From this study one can measure (choose one):

    A. The risk of acquiring Salmonellosis from pet turtles

    B. The prevalence of Salmonellosis in King County

    C. The incidence of Salmonellosis in King County

    D. The prevalence of pet turtles among Salmonellosis cases in King County

17. Analysis of data from a census of the population of a town in Georgia revealed a greater frequency of people reporting their age as being some multiple of the number 5 than any other. This is an example of: I. observer bias; II. respondent bias; III. digit preference; IV. random error.

    A. I and IV are correct

B. II and III are correct
C. II, III, and IV are correct
D. II and IV are correct

18. The following data set emanated from an epidemiological investigation of a disease outbreak eventually identified as being caused by staphylococcal intoxication, with turkey serving as the vehicle. Children and adults were affected similarly.

Illness Attack Rate by Time of Eating

Time of Eating (P.M.)	Number Interviewed	Number Ill	Attack Rate (%)
5:30	13	0	0
6:00	24	0	0
6:30	11	0	0
7:00	12	6	50
7:30	14	9	64
8:00	7	6	86
Total	81	21	26

Which of the following interpretations of these data fits best:
A. Dose-response effect
B. Ascertainment effect
C. Selection-bias effect
D. Digit-preference effect

19. What type of study was this?
A. Case series
B. Case-control
C. Prevalence
D. None of the above

20. During March and April, 1976, practicing physicians in West Ho Hum, Wyoming, reported an unusual number of new cases of diabetes mellitus among school children. The resident epidemiologist calculated that the incidence rate among school children for the two-month period was 5 per 10,000, which exceeded the endemic level by 500 percent. Five hundred children attended school in West Ho Hum, Wyoming. A wave of epidemic epimyositis swept through the community during February and March, 1976. Choose one of the following:
A. This situation should be classed as pandemic
B. The usual incidence of juvenile-onset diabetes mellitus in West Ho Hum during March and April is one case
C. The preceding epidemic produced metabolic decompensation in children who had impending diabetes
D. This is ridiculous

Answers to Specimen Examination Questions

1. *D*. These data resulted from testing a single blood specimen taken at a point in time for antibody to *T. Gondii*.

2. *A*. A glance at the figures in the row labeled "All ages" reveals a similar proportion of positives for men and women. However, the proportions positive by age are quite dissimilar, and therefore rates should be adjusted for age.

3. *C*. The study obviously is a prevalence study. No inferences concerning incidence or risk can be drawn from prevalence data.

4. *C*. Given the choice of answers to this question, all but *C* can be excluded perfunctorily. A cohort effect inherently distorts cross-sectional data. In this instance, the older people may have a higher prevalence because they were infected when young, during a time when the eskimo diet included more inadequately cooked flesh of marine mammals than at a later time. Antibody acquired early in life would persist indefinitely. On the other hand, the higher prevalence among older persons could have resulted from a longer period of exposure to a relatively low-level exposure, leading to a cumulative effect.

5. *D*. Hypothyroidism apparent at birth obviously had its onset sometime during gestation. Birth marks a point in time at which the condition becomes manifest, but it does not correspond to onset.

6. *C*. For every 6,000 births, one case could be identified if the test were 100 percent sensitive. However, the test only identified half of the cases that actually exist. Therefore, 12,000 live newborns would have to be tested to detect one case, and 120,000 to find ten cases.

7. *D*. See the fifth sentence in the problem statement.

8. *B*. By definition, treatment of early asymptomatic disease to prevent subsequent disability (cretinism) constitutes secondary prevention.

9. *A*. It would be difficult, if not impossible, to convince stewards of the public treasury to organize and fund a vast program with only half of the cases detectable by test and no indication of how many false positive cases would accrue.

10. *B*. With constant duration but decreasing incidence shown in the graph, the prevalence inevitably would decrease. The case fatality ratio, estimated by dividing mortality rates by incidence rates, would increase in proportion to the decrease in incidence when mortality is constant, as shown by the graph.

11. *C*. Assuming that both groups were exposed to the same extent, then both the vaccine group and the placebo group should have had virtually identical incidence rates. By definition the protection rate is the rate

of disease in the placebo group minus the rate in the vaccinated group divided by the rate in the placebo group; this quotient is then multiplied by 100 to convert the proportion into a percentage. The rate in the vaccine group was 10.8 per 100, and the rate in the placebo group was 20.1 per 100. Thus, the protection rate is:

$$\frac{20.1 - 10.8}{20.1} \times 100 = 46\%$$

12. *D.* The key sentence in this question is: "The levels of cholesterol in the two aliquots from each of the 50 specimens were then compared." This indicates that the intent of the study was to determine whether the test would yield reproducible results. Reproducibility and reliability are synonymous.

13. *A.* Validity, by definition, pertains to test accuracy, that is, how closely the test result approximates the true concentration of what is being measured.

14. *C.* Putting the data in a two-by-two table format helps solve this problem.

Used Reserpine	Cases	Controls
Yes	15	30
No	18	67
Total	33	97

By subtraction, the number of cases not exposed was 18 and the number of controls not exposed was 67. With these numbers inserted in the table, one can compute the relative risk as follows:

$$\frac{15 \times 67}{18 \times 30} = 1.86$$

15. *A.* Only cases are used to identify a possible determinant of Salmonellosis transmission in this instance.

16. *D.* The situation described does not permit any inferences about rate of disease, but rather the prevalence of a trait, that is, possession of a pet turtle.

17. *B.* In this circumstance, the preference for stating age as some multiple of five is obviously also a manifestation of respondent bias. Requesting actual date of birth is one way to circumvent this sort of bias.

18. *A.* Staphylococcal food poisoning is caused by ingestion of a toxin that is produced by the bacteria. The bacteria grow and produce the toxin

when the contaminated food provides an environment with the proper nutrients, moisture, pH, and temperature. The longer the contaminated turkey, which presumably was not refrigerated, remained uneaten, the more toxin it contained. Hence, the increasing attack rate with the lateness of the hour reflects an increased rate in association with an increased dose of toxin.

19. *D*. This was a nonconcurrent prospective study.

20. *D*. How many of the 500 children in the community would have had to have diabetes for the rate to be 5 per 10,000 during the two-month period?

Key Words and Phrases

About the Authors

Donald R. Peterson, a native of the Pacific Northwest, has devoted the bulk of his professional career to epidemiologic practice, research, and teaching. He received the M.D. from the University of Oregon and the M.P.H. from the University of California at Berkeley. Dr. Peterson served as epidemiologist for the Seattle-King County Department of Public Health for over a decade before joining the faculty as professor in the Department of Epidemiology at the University of Washington in Seattle. In 1976 he was appointed chairman of the Department. He has also served as visiting lecturer in the Department of Social and Preventive Medicine, Faculty of Medicine, University of Malaya, at Kuala Lumpur, Malaysia, from 1974 to 1975.

David B. Thomas received the M.D. from the University of Washington and the Dr.P.H. from Johns Hopkins University. He has also been a member of the faculty in departments of epidemiology at both of these institutions, and is currently associate professor at the University of Washington. He has taught courses in epidemiologic methods and cancer epidemiology. His research activities have involved investigations of infectious diseases, including studies of smallpox in the Indian subcontinent, and epidemiologic studies of various cancers.